Stacy
Garton

Finding the
"CAN"
in Cancer

*Provided as an educational resource
for your patients, courtesy of*

 Bristol-Myers Squibb

DISCLAIMER

This book is intended to provide supplemental information to those suffering with cancer, interested parties, families and friends. It is not intended as a replacement for professional advice. It is offered with the understanding that the authors are not engaged in rendering medical or other professional services. The use of information in this book is at the reader's discretion. The authors specifically disclaim any and all liability arising directly or indirectly from the use or application of any information contained in this book. If medical advice or other expert assistance is required, the service of a competent professional should be sought.

Finding the "CAN" in Cancer

For current oncology updates please visit

www.findingthecanincancer.com

Contents

Contents

Contents

Contents

Contents

Contents

Foreword

Battling cancer with an optimistic and upbeat attitude is a challenging task. It helps to have friends; particularly friends who know what you are up against. This book is many things: a pragmatic and practical handbook on dealing with the details of cancer treatment; a book with helpful and inspirational vignettes; and most of all, a story of friends. And not just any friends, but four friends who have faced all that a cancer diagnosis can entail, from standard chemotherapy and surgery to amputation and bone marrow transplant. I have had the honor and privilege of knowing each of them, and participating in some of their battles. Each exemplifies a depth of resourcefulness and optimism that has sustained them through the roughest of times. They have come together to write this book as a guide to "Finding the CAN in Cancer." It contains valuable advice garnered from years of experience facing this disease. Through this book, they have extended their love and friendship to others now facing this challenge. I know that those who read this book will find that love and friendship, and will be encouraged to thrive as they handle their own cancer ordeal.

P. Kelly Marcom, MD

Assistant Professor of Medicine

Director, Breast Medical Oncology and Hereditary Cancer Clinic

Duke University Multidisciplinary Breast Program

Prologue

Our book began simply as an attempt to pass along some tips for dealing with cancer to others who might be facing the same challenge. We gathered initially in the treatment room at the hospital, working while one or more of us received chemotherapy. Eventually, we graduated to home meetings, which became so much fun that often we got very little accomplished other than eating wonderful meals and laughing boisterously. Sometimes we wore silly hats, feather boas and other adornments; other times we simply "came as we were." We overcame many obstacles in the writing and came to view this as a metaphor for all that challenged us in our lives.

One especially difficult, yet amazing, meeting occurred several years ago now, when we gathered at a relative's home for an intensive three-day weekend – no families, no phones, no other responsibilities. And as it turned out, no plumbing! The weekend began with everyone arriving in the foyer greeted by the sight of toilet paper packages, which our hostess had thoughtfully left for us. We all agreed that it was foreshadowing (Susan even captured the moment with a photograph!). For the next three days, we endured overflowing toilets, a backed up septic tank, no flushing, sanitary clean-up crews and more. Probably worst of all, our computer crashed, resulting in our losing every bit of the work that we had labored over so diligently up to then. Other people probably would have quit, screamed, cried, or at the very least, yelled obscenities. But our group could not be deterred by such puny challenges. After all, we were dealing with a much bigger one - ongoing cancer treatments for three of us. One thing that cancer can do is put life into sharp focus. We laughed more that weekend than at any other time in our lives and became as close as people can become who must share such intimacies. We decided that the book was secondary to the wonder and joy of such a powerful communion of spirits.

This book is not intended as a work of fine literature, though we certainly hope it is readable, informative, and in some ways compelling. We are real people who have faced real challenges, speaking in our own words. We share our experiences in the hope of connecting with others undergoing similar challenges.

If we can convey one thing to you through this book, let it be this: love will sustain you during your difficulties as it did us that weekend. Along the way, in reading, we hope you will also find some things to help guide you on your cancer journey. This is our attempt to walk beside you, to offer you comfort, hope and most of all, love.

OUR STORIES

It's not the years in your life that count;
It's the life in your years.

-Abe Lincoln

Nancy

Take a trip with me on a cancer journey that has spanned over 20 years, and I hope you will find encouragement and hope along the way. Each patient's path is unique; I have learned that you can't compare your case to another case because no one has ever been created like you, and no one ever will be – not even if cloning becomes viable in the future. You are unique, and how you face challenges in life and respond to those challenges is unique to you. You are not a statistic! I have always taken the approach that if statistics say there is a one in 100 chance for survival, the other 99 might as well move over, because I am heading for the winning position at the finish line!

I also believe that there are two "B's" in facing any challenge we have in our lives. We can "B"come better or we can "B"come bitter. I happen to think that it is better to become better. The choice we make will make all the difference in how we handle our life's challenges; in how we respond to treatment; in how we respond to friends and family; in how they respond to us; and in how we respond to the negative feelings we may have, or to those negative thoughts that others unintentionally put into our minds. As you read this and you learn about some of my ups and downs, always keep in mind that I have made it through the rain, and am still making it through; and you can, too. There are so many new treatment options available today that were not available when I began my cancer journey. Had some of those options been available to me when I was diagnosed over 20 years ago, my journey may have been different. But, I can truthfully say that cancer has been a healing experience for my life, so I would not have changed it. My faith has been strengthened through the experience. It is much more important to be healed than to be cured. Many people are perfectly healthy, but they don't have a healed life. As a person strives to heal her life, an interesting thing happens: the immune system is also strengthened.

From the moment I was born, I was in the line of fire. The first time I ever became aware of cancer was when I learned that my maternal aunt had been diagnosed with breast cancer; a few years later another maternal aunt received the diagnosis. Although only five percent of breast cancers are inherited, I always knew that this and other factors put me in the high-risk category. Even with that information, I think I tried to deny that breast cancer was happening to me. Although my cancer journey officially began in 1982, I need to back up to a July morning in 1979 to give you the entire picture. At the age of 39, I was moving on with my life. One morning, as I was dressing for work, I noticed a dimple on my breast that I had not seen before. I always wanted dimples as a child, but I certainly never expected to see one on my breast! I had read that dimpling on the breast was a cancer warning sign, so I immediately made an appointment to see my gynecologist. He ordered a mammogram, and after examining me, he said, "Nancy, there is nothing to palpate, and the mammogram doesn't show anything; so you don't have a thing to worry about. Just watch it, and if you notice any changes, let me know." I breathed a sigh of relief, but knowing that I had several risk factors, which included a family history, I should have followed that still small voice within which kept saying to me, "Nancy, you should get another opinion." I wish I had followed that inner guidance, but instead I rationalized that surely if my doctor thought there were a problem he would have sent me to someone to get another opinion. I went merrily on my way in denial because I didn't notice any change for over two years. I had taken a new job which was very stressful and required lots of travel, so I put my health on the back burner.

In 1982, I noticed that the skin around the dimple was puckering, so off I went to see my gynecologist again. When he examined me this time he said, "Nancy, I'm afraid you may have breast cancer." I was stunned! When I left the doctor's office, I was reeling from the shock of hearing the word "cancer" related to me. My first thought was that if this were breast cancer, I didn't even know what to ask to make sure I was getting the best treatment. I remembered reading about the National Cancer Hotline (1-800-4CANCER). The National Cancer Institute sponsors this line for cancer patients and physicians to use to obtain information about cancer. I called them, and I found a

7

very caring and informed stranger on the other end of the phone. She gave me a list of questions to ask on my next visit to the surgeon whom the gynecologist had made an appointment for me to see. These questions would help me determine if I would be getting the best treatment. I knew that if this were cancer, it most likely had been there three years before, and I should seek the best place I could find to obtain treatment. After talking to the local surgeon and asking him some of the questions I had on my list, I realized that I needed to get to a comprehensive cancer center because at that time, the local doctor could not provide what I needed to fight the disease. I think anyone who faces a cancer diagnosis should always get a second opinion, because you don't get a second chance to get that second opinion. If you proceed, and then later find that you are not receiving the best treatment for your situation, you can't erase what has been done. What if a mistake has been made on the pathology report, and it isn't even cancer? Any good doctor will be comfortable with having you seek another opinion.

When I arrived at the Comprehensive Cancer Center, my surgical oncologist did a needle biopsy, which confirmed my worst fears. Yes, it was cancer! I remember walking out of the clinic, looking at other people going busily about their lives, and I was thinking, "How can life be going on as usual when I am facing this crisis?" It was almost surreal. I had a modified radical mastectomy and learned that I had 6 out of 19 positive lymph nodes. I didn't fully comprehend what all of that meant at the time, but I've learned a lot about cancer since that day, and

I learned that this put me at higher risk for a recurrence. One learns a new vocabulary when faced with cancer. My doctor scheduled adjuvant chemotherapy since the cancer had spread to the lymph system, and after seven chemotherapy treatments, which were administered every three weeks, I went on with my life. In 1982, there was very little they could do to combat nausea, but I am happy to say that the treatment of cancer has advanced over 20 years, and now, few patients experience nausea from chemotherapy. New drugs have been developed for that purpose. Also, new drugs have been developed to help boost the blood counts, leading to fewer infections in cancer patients.

I continued to have regular check-ups, always hoping that cancer was behind me. Three years after my mastectomy, I had my annual bone scan, and it revealed that the cancer had spread to my spine. I couldn't believe it! Stage 4! Statistics for my survival were 2 years. That was 17 years ago! I felt that my life and the cancer were out of control. Hearing the cancer had recurred was more difficult for me than hearing the original diagnosis. I sat down on my sofa and said, "God, I am out of control! Please give me something to help me get through this." I opened the Bible, and these words were staring back at me: "My peace I give you. Let not your heart be troubled, and neither let it be afraid." Wow! That's the message I needed to calm my fears and give me the peace I needed to face the new challenge. When I closed my eyes to say thanks, I received another wonderful message. I saw in my mind's eye a huge billboard with giant black letters that spelled the word "cancer." As I was wondering what kind of message this was, my eyes just focused on the first three letters of that big black word...CAN! Yes, the first three letters of the word 'CANcer' spell CAN! I had been fighting cancer for three years and had seen that word many times, but I had never seen the CAN in CANcer. I have shared that story with many people and have yet to meet the first one who has seen the CAN. It was a message to me... "You CAN survive!"..." You CAN help others"... "You CAN make a difference." That CAN message has helped me on this 20-year plus cancer journey. I began my new treatment armed with a "CAN" attitude, trying to bounce back from the shock of another bout with cancer. I had six weeks of radiation treatments to my spine. I was anxious about it as most people are when starting a radiation treatment, but the people in the treatment area were wonderful, and they helped to allay my fears. It took longer to get up onto the treatment table than it did to have the radiation.

When I completed the radiation, I started taking a hormone therapy called tamoxifen, which had just been approved for breast cancer treatment. For eight years I was considered a "NED"...no evidence of disease, and my hopes were high that now cancer was in my past. In 1993, another bone scan and another shock...the cancer was on the march down my spine again. Now, what would we do? Making decisions about treatment is one of the most difficult challenges on the cancer journey. I have been blessed with wonderful, caring doctors who have considered me a partner in the decision-making process. Although I have been on some type of treatment since

1985, I have had a very good quality of life, and until recently, I have been able to work at a demanding job. The important thing is that I have survived and thrived. It would take an entire book to write about each treatment I have received, so I will sum the treatments up by saying that I have had over 14 types of chemotherapy or hormone therapy, 12 surgical procedures, 12 weeks of radiation therapy, and more bone scans, CT scans, MRIs, PET scans and other scans than I could count.

When possible, I feel that it is important for me to participate in trials on new drugs and treatments when I can because this helps the research community develop new drugs and treatments for cancer. I feel fortunate to have participated in a Phase I Trial of a new vaccine being developed and I was the eighth person to receive it. They used my own dendritic cells to make the vaccine and then supercharged the cells and gave them back to me in an IV infusion. While I was on the trial they proved with my case that they could actually stimulate one's own immune system to fight the cancer. NBC Nightly News interviewed me to tell the nation about this new, promising cancer treatment, which had no side effects. Similar vaccines are now being explored at many research institutions across the country and the National Cancer Institute has had some fantastic results using a vaccine to treat melanoma patients. I pray that one day these will prove effective, and we will have such treatments available to fight all cancers. The cancer journey has been like a roller coaster ride…up and down and holding on for dear life. We continue to use new drugs; some of them have been effective, and some have not. The lesson for me is never to give up hope, and to remember when a door closes, a window opens. I have always looked at each window as a window of opportunity. I have also learned that a sense of humor is invaluable and can help one cope with many situations. Because one of the chemotherapies I was taking completely destroyed my tear ducts, using eye makeup became a real challenge, especially when I lost my eyelashes and eyebrows. The water, which was naturally produced by my eyes, had no drainage system; and it washed off my creative efforts at putting on eyeliner. Because the chemotherapy caused neuropathy in my fingers and the loss of some of my fingernails, using false eyelashes was a real challenge since it was difficult to do intricate things like putting on false eyelashes. One day I had to speak at a luncheon, which was being held at an exclusive country club, and I decided if there was ever a time to wear false eyelashes, this was it! Knowing that they might wash right off my eyes, I warned my colleagues that if they should see something black and furry lying on my cheek, not to swat it off because it would probably be a false eyelash that had floated off, not an insect. Waterproof eyeliner and mascara have been a great help with the eye makeup dilemma. Beautiful lessons come to me in the most unexpected ways. One day, I was starting a new chemotherapy treatment, which was going to be pretty tough. My nurse came by to start the infusion, and she said, "Nancy, look outside. We are having a terrible storm." I turned to look out, and the sky was dark. It was pouring rain, and the wind was blowing so hard the trees were bending to the breaking point. When I turned back and looked around the room, I saw many cancer patients who were facing storms in their lives. After a while the nurse came back and said that the storm was over. When I looked outside this time, I saw a giant, vivid rainbow outside the window. My heart filled with gratitude as I realized that a rainbow is a sign of hope, and I felt that this was a good omen as I started that new treatment. When I was having an MRI in 1993 to confirm that the cancer had spread in my spine, I had earphones and could listen to music. As I was lying there thinking about how serious this new diagnosis was for me, a song came flooding into my head with a powerful message - Mariah Carey's song, "Heroes"©. I knew when I heard it that this was a message sent from God that I would be fine. The lyrics included these words:

"And then a hero comes along with the strength to carry on, and you cast your fears aside, and you know you CAN survive. So when you feel like hope is gone, look inside you and be strong, and you'll finally see the truth - that a hero lies in you." Yes, there is a hero inside each of us; we just need to discover that when we are facing challenges.

My dear friend, the late Bob Stone, decided to start a team to help him face his challenge with cancer. I decided to follow his lead and start a team to help cheer me on to victory. I identified friends and family whom I thought would keep me in their prayers, and nine years ago I sent out my first newsletter to ask that they join the team. That song gave me the name of my team...The Team of Heroes. I liked that because heroes save lives and inspire courage. This team has been very important to me on my cancer journey. Over 400 people all across the nation cheer me on with encouraging notes and messages, and they pray for me on a regular basis. Heroes are all around us, but the important hero is the one that lies inside each of us. We never know how much courage and strength we have until we are put to the test. One of my doctors said that the medicine he gives is not nearly as important as what is inside the patient – the attitude, the will to fight, the active involvement a patient maintains when seeking treatment decisions and the determination to survive. When I asked my doctor about a new drug I had heard about, he e-mailed me to say, "Don't mean to be discouraging, but this new drug is not the magic bullet. But then you have your own magic bullet. We just need to figure out what it is so we can share it with every other woman who has breast cancer." I have given you some of those magic bullets in this story, and I hope you will use them. Great medical care is one of the bullets used in my arsenal of weapons to fight cancer. I have also incorporated other complementary modalities in my treatment: meditation, prayer, visualization, healing touch therapy, laughter, herbs, and self-hypnosis. Some of the best medical centers in the country are integrating complementary medicine in their treatment options. Exercise is very important to help strengthen the bones and to prevent stress fractures. Unfortunately, I have always been sedentary and have not considered exercise the favorite way to use my time…although I certainly wish I had. So, take a lesson from me and consult a physical therapist to help you determine the best exercise plan for your situation. Although the cancer has spread to my skull, clavicle, several ribs, almost every vertebra from the top of my spine to the bottom, both femurs, pelvic bones, both arms, the liver and lungs, I am leading a good life. Treatment has become a part of my life, and I have learned to live with that. I've found that you can put "treat" into treatment when you have dear friends and family to accompany you and make it a pleasant experience. The nurses who administer my chemotherapy are terrific. My friend, Pam, who is one of the co-authors of this book, always brings flowers when I have treatment, and she and I have spent countless hours laughing and catching up on what is happening in the world and with each other. Those beautiful flowers brighten my life and the lives of the nurses and other patients having treatment because all of us can enjoy the beauty of her garden and creativity.

My faith helps me withstand the storms in my life. My husband, family and friends have been beside me supporting me every step of the way, and their support makes all the difference as I continue to go down the long and winding road on a cancer journey, one that has truly healed my life.

Nancy Weaver Emerson

Pam

My personal, intimate involvement with cancer goes back over twenty-five years, although it was not my own, but that of my close family members. My paternal grandmother was diagnosed with pancreatic cancer some twenty years ago, and my father-in-law had prostate cancer for many years. I was a caregiver for him during much of that time, going with him to surgeries and helping with his post-op and supportive care. It was during this time that I began to try to deal with all of the symptoms which accompany cancer and which can make day-to-day life such a challenge. I observed that many times it is the so-called "little" problems that can cause the most difficulties in everyday life (this is true emotionally as well as physically). I tried to become a problem solver for lots of these troubling side effects of disease and treatment and was delighted to be able to help in some small ways to make life more comfortable for him. One of the things I remember most vividly, for example, was how distressed he was with the small cuts on the ends of his fingers, a result of one of his chemotherapy drugs. I was thrilled to be able to solve that miserable little problem for him by telling him about liquid bandage (NewSkin®, tissue glue, etc.), which made him as pleased as anything I could have done for him other than offer him a complete cure!

My father, in the years after my father-in-law's diagnosis, underwent several major surgeries to replace both knees, both hips, and one hip for a second time! He had all these operations performed at the medical center in my city so that I could help my mother nurse him and be a support to them both. It was during one of his immediate post-op periods that my mother learned of her endometrial cancer. She had recently had an endometrial biopsy, and although she had not received a report from that procedure, she had forgotten it since she was focusing on helping my father. She made a very wrong assumption: that everything is fine if you don't hear from the doctor's office following a procedure. (A good tip: if you don't hear from the doctor's office within a week, call the doctor and ask for the report!) Several weeks passed, and my mother's elderly father died unexpectedly. The day before his funeral, she received a call from her physician telling her that they had accidentally overlooked her pathology report, that she had endometrial cancer, and that she needed to have a total hysterectomy immediately. During these difficult times for my parents, I nursed them simultaneously, and we all dealt with the grief of my grandfather's death. Fortunately, my mother recovered well and required no further treatment at that time. The following Christmas, however, she suffered a total bowel obstruction, probably as a result of adhesions from her cancer surgery. She and my father again stayed with us so that I could care for them. All of these difficult times afforded me wonderful opportunities to learn many very practical things about how to care for patients at home and in the hospital. One of the best things to come from this adversity, though, was the priceless gift of time it afforded me to share with my parents, and I would not have traded that for anything. My husband and our three children also served as caregivers, and as a result, these four doctors know firsthand about what happens to patients after they leave the hospital.

Some years after my father-in-law's death, I cared for his wife, my mother-in-law, for eight years after her diagnosis with colon cancer. During that challenging time, I learned about cancer in the most "up close and personal" ways as I accompanied her on all her visits to the doctor, treatments and surgeries and helped with every aspect of her personal care. Again, I was called upon to be a problem solver for all of the difficulties of living with cancer. By the time of her death several years ago, I had acquired quite a store of tips and helpful advice about things that can make this path a smoother one.

One of the greatest blessings of my life has been my friendship with Nancy Emerson, and through her, with Susan and Terri. The story of this amazing relationship is dramatic and still awe-inspiring to me. I knew Nancy as a patient with cancer, and our paths crossed several times over a period of years. I would always think and say, "We need to get together, to know each other better." She would agree, but then as often happens, time and circumstance would river us apart. One summer I happened to see her at my mother-in-law's treatment, and we said the usual things and drifted apart once again. In the fall of that same year, I had a dramatic dream in which I knew that I had to call Nancy immediately! The next morning I did just that, explained my dream and asked if we could meet as soon as possible. I knew with the greatest of certainty that God was calling us to be friends. She agreed, and we began really getting to know each other. One wonderful opportunity to do this was at her treatments, which sometimes can take several hours at a time. I began to accompany her to these sessions and looked forward to them with great anticipation because they provided us with the gift of time to get to know each other in a way that we would not have otherwise. I could write an entire book about the blessings that have come from my time and friendship with Nancy. We never have enough time to finish talking, and since we always laugh and share so much at these sessions, we have begun calling that time our "TREATment," rather than "treatment." It was at the treatment center that I met Susan and Terri, my amazing and wonderful friends, who volunteer there.

Immediately following the final days of my mother-in-law's difficult and courageous struggle with her cancer, I was diagnosed with endometrial cancer-in-situ, which is the earliest stage of the disease. As I told my three friends, "Some people will do anything to belong to a group!" I had a total hysterectomy several months after diagnosis and have not had to undergo any further treatment. When I first heard the news that I had cancer, I was stunned. It is a very human reaction, I think, that we deal with difficult things all the time and yet are so surprised when they affect us personally! As a result of all my experience with my family's illnesses and Nancy's, I did not fear cancer the way I might have otherwise. Instead, I approached it as a problem and proceeded to do what needed to be done to take care of it. I have been fortunate to have needed no further treatment at this time, and I do not think about that possibility except when I go in for my follow-up appointments. If I have to face this problem again, I trust that I have learned from my friends to approach it with strength and grace as they have done. I believe that as we face any challenge in life, it is not so much what we have to deal with but how we deal with it that matters. In some ways, I don't feel worthy to be in the same group with these three remarkable women, my friends; but we do share a common struggle: dealing with cancer, whether as a caregiver or a care receiver.

Pamela Davis Leight

Susan

I bear a strong resemblance to my mother, but I would have to attribute my love of reading to my dad. He always had a book going and especially loved a good "whodunit." Although I am the same way, I haven't enjoyed having an aura of mystery surrounding my medical history. I was first diagnosed with cancer in 1979. In the years since then, I have dealt with both recurrences and a new diagnosis. I have had two types of cancer, but the primary site for both remains unknown. I guess you could say that we have never located the "smoking gun."

In December, 1979, I was 34 years old. Our children were ages six, nine and eleven, and my husband George had just accepted a job promotion relocating us to South Florida. Upon discovering a small lump on the side of my chest wall under my right arm, I had a biopsy, which revealed an "undifferentiated malignant carcinoma," but the site of origin was unknown. Ironically, I previously had a benign lump removed, in nearly the same location, one year to the day. My reaction to being told I had cancer was not uncommon. It was basically – "oh no, this can't be happening to me." Up until that time life had not just been good, it had been great - a supportive and loving husband, three healthy and wonderful kids, and we had even had the opportunity to do a four- year assignment in France. I now look back on that as the "Hallmark" phase of life. It had a greeting card quality to it. Then reality entered the scene. After extensive diagnostic tests, it was determined that I most probably had early stage breast cancer, and I had a modified mastectomy followed by six weeks of radiation. The pathology reports following surgery never revealed a specific type of cancer conclusively. During this early stage, I went through phases of denial, pity, and times of being mad and then sad. However, I also was guided in learning some important lessons. First and foremost, I learned to appreciate the good things I had in my life. My husband, family and friends, my faith and an ever-increasing awareness of God's presence in my life were lifelines to me. I also had a lesson in the importance of laughter courtesy of our youngest. We had been very open with the kids regarding my illness. We tried to give them age-appropriate information and to prepare them as best we could for what would be happening. This was over 20 years ago, and since a lot less was done on an outpatient basis then, there were numerous hospitalizations. We had explained radiation treatments as a hi-tech process that would get rid of Mommy's bad cells. I arranged my treatments for mid-morning, having discovered early in the game that if you have a heartbeat you still qualify to drive carpool. When Michael, then six, arrived home from school the day of my first treatment, all I had to show for my hi-tech encounter were several ink marks on my skin showing the treatment field. He was quite impressed with this, especially since he had frequently been told that he was never to put marker on his skin. I explained things as best I could and left to pick up his older sister. When I returned home, I discovered that he had assembled four little buddies so he could show them my

24

markings. I once again launched into my explanation, and they soon went off to his room. I settled down to a cup of tea, thinking I had taken care of that. Within a short time, the merry little band reappeared covered in magic marker designs and announced that they weren't going to wash theirs off until I could wash mine off! All I could do was burst out laughing: this whole cancer thing definitely had its unexpected twists.

Life settled down to a "normal" routine once again, and I became quite convinced that this illness was all behind me. But such was not the case. About 16 months later, I developed pressure under my arm. After more tests and biopsies, I was diagnosed with a recurrence, but again indefinite as to what type of cancer. Pathology reports were sent to several centers, and we consulted with different doctors, most of whom were baffled, some of whom were just discouraging. I had a terrific family doctor who said that we would keep pursuing the diagnosis. The hardest part was the uncertainty. There was no consensus as to what type of cancer I had and how to treat it. I had always thought of medicine as being black and white, very definitive. I was learning that is not always the case, and it was a hard lesson. I found myself worrying about all the things that might happen and where it might spread. One specialist I consulted said that based on how the disease was progressing, he felt there was very little that could be done (remember this was over 20 years ago), and most likely, my life expectancy was about 18 months. Processing information of that nature can happen in a strange way. As George and I walked out of the office, my first comment was, "Did you see that he was wearing cowboy boots? How dare someone in boots tell me I am going to die?" To be honest, I don't have anything against cowboy boots, but it was the only fragment of the situation that I could deal with at the moment. We then met with another physician, and I was told that my best chance for survival was to have a forequarter amputation, which is the removal of my arm, shoulder, clavicle and top ribs. The tumor had spread into the axilla and was close to invading the lung. This scenario had never appeared in all my "what ifs," and perhaps that is just as well, because it seemed hard to imagine. The surgeon who proposed this course of action is a special physician with whom I am still in touch. I remember saying to him, – "Can I live like that?" and he remarked, "Think about that question, 'if you can live like that.' Having you live is what it is all about." With his encouragement, we went to another cancer center for a consultation and were once again told that the amputation was the best option. How do you prepare yourself for limb loss and disfigurement? I am not sure you truly can. I tried to stay focused on the reasons I wanted to live and asked God to please give me the strength to deal with all the other challenges that were going to come my way. I was right-handed, and it was my right arm that was being amputated. I was about to turn 36, and I was going to have to relearn how to write my name. It was hardly the activity of choice for this stage in my life. Once again I learned an important lesson from one of my children. Having been a psychology major, I felt that I was putting my lessons to good use and doing well handling discussions with the children. I was doing most of my crying in the shower or behind closed doors. One night, as I was tucking our 11-year-old daughter into bed, I told her it was okay to cry or to be mad about all of this, and that she didn't have to hide it. She looked up at me and very quietly said, "It would be a lot easier for me to cry if you would let me see you cry once in a while"... so much for college psychology. Needless to say, we had a good cry together. The surgery went well, and I slowly worked my way through the recovery. I really didn't think a lot about the cancer at this stage. I decided that having paid this high a price to beat this thing, I was just going to focus on getting through it. Adjusting to limb loss is every bit as much a mental as it is a physical adjustment. Physically there was the challenge of learning to do things with my left hand only, and then I had to come to a level of acceptance of how I looked. When I was younger it had been very important to me that I fit in, and yet I never really felt that I did. Now I was dealing with a unique shape, and to my surprise, I found it to be quite freeing. I threw the word "normal" out of my vocabulary and began to be comfortable with being me and accepting that it was an ever-changing experience. About two years later, I developed a severe infection in the material that had been placed in my chest wall to protect the lung from where the ribs were missing. I was starting to feel as if I were on a warranty plan that had a two-year recall. Weeks of IV treatment, rushed trips to the hospital, and two major surgeries (one lasting for ten hours) ensued, but the cancer did not recur. However, I developed a healthy respect for the fact that cancer isn't the only thing that can make you sick; meanwhile the children were becoming very resilient to schedule disruptions. One night I spiked a fever and had to go to the hospital in the middle of the night. We woke the kids up because we had promised them that we would always keep them informed of what was going on, which was appropriate since they were now 10, 13 and 15, respectively. We explained the situation, took a family vote, and decided they could have a "go to school late" pass. As we were leaving, our oldest daughter was taking charge and helping the others to make some kind of fancy concoctions in the blender. She reasoned that if they were up that late, they might as well do something exciting. We were all learning to look for fun in the midst of strange events.

For the next 15 years, I was closely watched and inspected, but except for some basal and squamous cell surface skin cancer, I remained cancer free. I had been given the gift of an extension of my life and an appreciation for how precious and fragile life is. Never going more than six months between visits to the oncologist helped me to keep things in perspective. Twenty years to the day after my first diagnosis, I again developed cancer. A biopsy of a small lump under the skin on the side of my cheek showed malignancy, not definitive as to type. Sound familiar? I had a parotidectomy, and no further cancer was detected. We were now living in North Carolina, and after studying my medical history, the doctors realized that I was a bit of a strange case. The surgery revealed no further malignancy, so we were really no closer to understanding what was happening. Four months later, a lump appeared under the scar tissue, and I had another parotidectomy. This time a nerve had to be removed, resulting in some paralysis to the side of my face. The pathology report on the tumor revealed that I had melanoma, which, because a primary site had never been detected on the skin, was categorized as metastatic. I was trying to adjust to the diagnosis and to the side effects of the surgery, and neither was an easy task. Some things get easier the more you do them, but I am not sure being told you have cancer is one of them. The treatment course we decided upon was six weeks of radiation treatment and seven months of vaccine immunotherapy involving one shot a month.

"Park the popcorn popper parallel to the pumpkin patch..." No, I haven't totally lost it, but that is what I walked around the house and drove to work saying. I was having trouble pronouncing certain letters, especially "p's" and again it helped to focus on this dimension of the situation rather than dwell on the diagnosis. I went to a speech therapist who did some research and told me that doing certain exercises with my mouth and rubbing my cheek with lemon Italian ice would help generate nerve growth. We were all quite anxious to see if I started talking with an Italian accent. I didn't, but we did take a trip to Italy last year, which was wonderful! There was a different aspect to my cancer experience this time, and that was my job. I have been fortunate enough to be working with a cancer patient support program for the past several years. Through this experience I have the opportunity and privilege to interact with many individuals dealing with cancer. Cancer is not meant to become an identity for any of us, but there is a bond among those who travel this road. Getting to know others facing the many challenges of this journey has given me great strength and inspiration, and I am immensely grateful to each of them and most especially to my dear friends with whom I have collaborated on this book. Looking back, I think that I knew from the start there would be other recurrences. Two years later I discovered a lump on my leg; it was surgically removed, and pathology showed I again had melanoma. Because it was in a different region of my body, I was diagnosed as having Stage IV metastatic melanoma. My daughter, who is an oncology nurse, was driving home with us from the doctor's appointment. I remember questioning her about how many cancer stages there are. "Just four, Mom," was her reply. Well, I didn't care for the sound of that. Did that mean I was supposed to contact the undertaker? How long could you drag out Stage IV? Could I reverse the order of this and drop back to Stage II? I was at the point where this was as much a mind game as it was a physical one. I had moments of feeling scared and overwhelmed, and then I would remember that I knew others who had Stage IV cancer, and they were still very much alive. It seems that for some of us being a cancer patient is a chronic condition.

I truly believe that God gives me the strength to deal with this one step at a time. I look upon my cancer as a chronic disease. There is always a certain undercurrent of anxiety about what will happen next, but there is also an appreciation of how special the here and now is. I heard a wonderful saying many years ago that I try to abide by, "dream as if you'll live forever, and live as if you won't." It saddens me to think that anyone has to have cancer, and yet it has been a part of my life for so long that I honestly don't know how my life would have transpired without it. It has certainly been difficult, and yet it has been the door to many blessings in my life. It has taught me lessons and assisted me in focusing on the truly important things in life. There are other ways to learn and experience these things, but for me cancer was the path my life took. My faith and my ever-increasing awareness of God's immense love for me have sustained me through difficult trials time and again. My husband has been a loving partner and an anchor for our family through it all; and I rejoice when I realize that our youngest was six when I was first diagnosed, and in the coming year, two of our six grandchildren will turn six-years-old. My blessings are too numerous to count. I am different now than I was twenty-four years ago. Then, I went to a physician looking to be told what to do. Now I have become an active participant in my treatment plan decisions. I believe in researching my options, and I practice complementary medicine as part of my wellness-plan. Some of this progression has been the result of my maturity, and another factor has been the increasing availability of information. There is a learning curve to being a cancer patient just as there is to all other experiences. Many of us have had to go it alone through that learning process; our hope is that

31

this book may help to smooth your way through some of the curves in your journey, those blind spots where it is hard to look ahead or to see behind.

We certainly don't claim to know it all, but we do hope that sharing what we have learned may be of some help. Please know that we wish to offer you not only the knowledge learned from our experiences, but a sense of companionship and encouragement. May you discover on the course of your journey strength, courage, and peace that will see you through.

Susan Comerford Moonan

Terri

The first thought I would like to share with you is gratitude. I want to thank God for guiding me through this challenge since 1989 which helped me to share the special life He has given me. There are so many family members, friends and acquaintances to thank for their genuine concern, kind words, positive thoughts and unending prayers.

Growing up in a rural town outside of New Orleans, I remember being a normal, healthy child with no major illnesses. I went to a Catholic school and taught guitar for more than ten years. My parents were divorced when I was 12 years old, and I seemed to cope well with being thrown into what was then known as a dysfunctional family. At 17, while planning my wedding, I discovered a mass in my left breast; I was relieved that the tumor was benign.. For the next eleven years, I never considered the possibility of having another tumor.

On the night prior to my first vacation cruise in 1989, I found a lump in my right breast; I was 28 years old. Let me preface this by saying that I had been under a tremendous amount of stress in the previous two years. I was experiencing a nasty divorce with a threatening custody battle, working a job while on 24-hour call; my sister lost her five-year-old son to a rare muscle disease; and I was a single mom with a very active six-year-old. The importance of reducing stress in your life is crucial; I believe it was a major contributor to the breakdown of my immune system.

33

I refused to cancel my much-needed vacation and decided to schedule an appointment with my doctor as soon as I returned from my trip.

In looking back, I made the right decision because it was on that vacation that I met Eric, the man I would soon marry. Eric was working aboard the cruise ship, and we were only able to see each other for six hours every Saturday. While waiting for my biopsy appointment, I received a call from my employer saying that there was a job opening in Houston, Texas; I leapt at the opportunity, knowing I could begin a new life with my daughter, Cassie, and reduce some stress in my life. I started packing for my move to Texas and had a breast biopsy the following week. The results were not what I expected. The tumor was malignant - and my life had forever changed. Within two weeks of finding the lump, I found out I had breast cancer, I had a new job in an unfamiliar city, and... I had met the man of my dreams. Having known Eric for only two weeks, I told him of my diagnosis; he supported my decision to get a mastectomy. To me, there was never an option to do anything else. There were no tears, just concern with the upcoming surgery. "Just tell me what needs to be done," was my reaction. I trusted my faith in God to pull me through such a traumatic event at such an early age. I believe that God carried me through and also answered my prayers when Eric came into my life. The modified radical mastectomy took place in New Orleans, and I was told that chemotherapy was not necessary. The doctor said I should find an oncologist in Houston and follow up in six months. Eric and I had a long distance relationship for six months, and I began my re-constructive surgery immediately after the move to Texas. My Mom would fly from Tennessee to be with me during each procedure and help with taking care of Cassie. I had a tissue expander placed got saline injections for eight weeks. My reconstruction was almost complete when I went for my six-month check-up. To my surprise, the oncologist suggested that I begin chemotherapy. I was initially told that chemotherapy was not necessary so I decided to get a second opinion. It was then that I learned the importance of second opinions. Eric had finished his commitment on the cruise ship and was with me when I went to find a new oncologist. We met with Dr. J. for our second opinion; he was just beginning his private practice after 13 years of specializing in breast cancer at MD Anderson Hospital in Houston. He didn't wait for me to decide if I would get the chemotherapy; he told me that I would be starting my chemo in two days and that he had already arranged for me to have a port-a-cath placed in my chest. When I think back on the techniques and toxicity of drugs in 1989, they seem so primitive today. It was a very foggy time in my life, but I remember vividly the first time I lost my hair. My dad and step-mom were visiting, and she had been my hairdresser for many years. Having her cut off all my hair was a traumatic time and we all shared a few tears that day. I remember praying that I would never have to watch my daughter experience such a devastating event. I took control of the situation as best I could which was to shave my head, but I couldn't control the fact that I felt as if I were losing a part of my identity with the loss of my hair. Since that first time, I have had to undergo the loss of my hair nine more times- it gets a little easier each time but it's not one of my favorite events- especially in the winter!

I have vague memories of Eric taking care of Cassie and sending her off to first grade, helping her with homework and being a fulltime dad. He stepped into our lives and accepted all the responsibilities with no prior parenting experience. He was there to hold my head over the toilet many days and nights and made sure that I took baths and ate regular meals. Because of the powerful drugs I took to keep me from vomiting, I would sleep continuously for three days following treatments. It was a difficult time to start a new relationship, but Eric was a special man who had true love for me, he was my knight in shining armor. We had "cancer free" days - once a week would go to see a movie or go fishing; we would do anything but talk about cancer or its side effects.

I chose to work during my chemo treatments; my generous employer compensated me with time and pay. I had a great boss who was very understanding and I consider one of my dearest friends today. I also had a new group of friends at work who supported me emotionally and physically at work. Although my immediate family lived six hours away, they traveled to be with me whenever possible; they also supported me with many daily phone calls. The significance of a support circle like this is immeasurably important in the recovery of your mental attitude and the subsequent effects it has on healing your physical body.

After six months, I completed chemotherapy and life returned to "normal." My hair grew back, and we went about our daily activities.

One year to the day after we met, and not a hair on my head, Eric got down on one knee and proposed marriage. We were married on December 1, 1990, a year-and-a-half after diagnosis. We went blissfully about our lives, and for the next seven years I was cancer free. We chose to live in extraordinary ways and did things most people only dream of doing. Cancer had definitely left its mark on our lives; we wanted to grab all the happiness and enjoyment that life has to offer. We traveled to exotic islands in foreign countries on scuba diving trips. Eric and I fulfilled a lifelong passion of flying; we bought a small airplane and got our private pilot licenses together. We experienced unusual events like getting to drive a US Navy nuclear submarine while visiting Eric's brother on a family excursion. We took a two-week train trip to the west coast and along the Canadian border so we could see the beautiful country in which we live. I went bungee jumping over the Guadalupe River in Texas; which was thrilling; as was white water rafting down the New River in West Virginia. If an exciting opportunity presented itself, we experienced it. We were working lots of hours at our jobs, but it was affording us our desired lifestyle. We built a house in a suburb of Houston, and I could see some stress starting to build in our lives. It was when we both decided to "jump off" the corporate ladder, quit our jobs and try to build a business for ourselves, that the stress cascaded and we ended up losing a lot of money instead. Cassie and Eric's step-relationship left a lot to be desired most of the time, and that became a constant battle among the three of us. As in any marriage, there are valleys and peaks, and we had our fair share - we just happened to have more valleys than peaks at this time in our lives. The financial stress was getting worse so we decided to take a job offered to Eric and move 1,200 miles to Durham, North Carolina.

The medical (HMO) plan at Eric's new job required me to have a baseline of tests when we arrived in North Carolina. Unbeknownst to me and after the baseline, a tumor grew in my lung untreated for 14 months (I guess someone dropped the ball). I found a pea-sized lump under my left arm, and had it biopsied. I have heard it said that blessings come in small packages, and I believe that small lump was mine. I was given a local block of anesthetic to biopsy the lump and subsequently had a slight pneumothorax (puncture to lung), which is common and mends itself in a couple days. However, I caught a virus and vomited for 24 hours, which caused the slight pneumothorax to collapse my left lung completely. I was told I needed a chest tube inserted (which should not be slighted as insignificant - it has been one of the most painful experiences of my cancer history). It was the good news/bad news scenario - the good news was that "it" had not grown much in the last 14 months… the bad new was obvious. There was my impending future all lit up on x-ray; it revealed a tumor in my lung, which was thought to be breast cancer metastasis. I was admitted into the hospital on that symbolically cold day in February 1997. After consulting with my oncologist and thoracic surgeon, we determined that it was the best time to remove the tumor since the chest tube was already in place. While exploring the area during surgery, the surgeon found that there were cancer cells in my pericardium (the sack around my heart.)

My life had taken a new and unusual turn into the world of medicine; this was not a career that I had chosen - it had been assigned! Thus began my education about cancer and living through an ordeal that was beyond comprehension at the time. I continued to receive chemotherapy for another year. My scan results were conclusive: the cancer was growing and new tumors were forming in my left lung.

The next challenge presented was a stem cell transplant, so I entered the bone marrow clinic in April 1998. There are many people who want to know about this experience, but for the most part, I don't remember many of the details, thanks to today's pharmaceutical advancement and good drugs (or as we call it, "better living through chemistry"). I do remember the last day of high dose chemotherapy in the hospital, it was a vivid memory my conscious mind surfaced through heavy drugs, and it occurred to me that this could be how dying would feel. Chemotherapy is designed to kill cells in your body, good and bad. That was the first time the thought of death ever crossed my mind. God stays with me at all times, and this was a time that I knew He was there. He carried me through those days of chemo, re-infusion of my stem cells and the weeks and months that followed. I also had my family next to me at such a crucial time in my life.

I have always had a high tolerance to pain and tend to bounce back quickly when knocked down from life's challenges, physical, mental or emotional. This was one of the toughest times that I can remember; I believed I would bounce back in five or six months, but I was humbled by my inability to achieve what before I had always been able to do. The next year was a struggle as I tried several new drugs.

I wanted to use the down time productively, and I began to plan our new home. It was a great time to research the project, and I needed another goal to keep pushing me forward. I became a general contractor during that time and began to build our house. One year after my stem cell transplant, tests revealed another growth on my lung, and I began chemotherapy immediately. I continued to focus on building our house and took breaks only when I needed to get a treatment. We moved into our new home ten months later, and building it was truly enjoyable.

I have experienced some form of drug therapy every week or so, since 1997. It has been my goal to outlive the 30% expectation of the prognosis given to me many years ago. My doctor has told me on repeated occasions that my treatment options were becoming limited, and I understand that it's about buying time with different drug combinations. This is part of the ultimate wait-and-see game. This so-called "game" has bought me many additional years of life.

Having exhausted the use of breast cancer drugs, my doctor tried lung cancer drugs to minimize or eliminate cell growth. The 15 different chemotherapies over the years have either stabilized the growth or done nothing to deter its growth. It was time to go back into surgery to remove the ever-growing tumors in my lung, as cells had spread throughout. I began chemo again and also started using the drug Iressa. Four months after starting this protocol, my scans came back cancer free. It was a great year for us but on my 44th birthday, a sarcoma was found in my abdomen, so I went back into surgery to have it removed. Prior to this discovery, my doctor wanted to do some genetic testing because of the unusual tumor reduction from Iressa. The results were conclusive that the breast cancer that was thought to be in my lungs was a primary lung cancer; the re-diagnosis of the pea-sized lump under my arm was a new primary breast cancer, and this sarcoma was yet another a primary cancer. I have been identified as having the Li-Fraumeni cancer gene.

Iressa's effectiveness is about two years and the tumors began to grow in my lung again. In the two years of remission, my treatment option cup was refilled. In mid-2006 we began a targeted therapy approach to treat the lung tumors with antibodies. For the most part, my chemotherapy has been replaced with antibody regimens. Since my clinic is at a research hospital, it gave us the opportunity to try different combinations. I began to take the antibody Tarceva and eight days later I began vomiting with severe headaches. A CT scan revealed a 2cm tumor on my brainstem. After being admitted to the hospital for an MRI, it showed that 90% of the tumor was hemorrhage. A small (mm) tumor in the occipital (visual) lobe was found and spots on my lower spine and scapula were found as well.

We speculate that the hemorrhage was a result of taking Tarceva. Again it was another blessing in disguise.

I was scheduled to begin 14 days of whole-head low-dose radiation, which is a treatment that I have managed to avoid in the previous years. A treatment that was also prescribed was SRS (stereotactic radio surgery). A halo is used to stabilize the head for the high dose targeted radiation to the tumor in my brain. Having this halo placed requires that it be screwed into your skull in four places. It was the four injections of anesthesia into my head, at the same time, that was the most challenging. It lit a fire in me to find alternative pre-medication methods to minimize the excruciating pain for future patients who must have this procedure. The radiation process is behind me and I have resumed taking the antibodies. A combination of two antibodies resulted in a rash that was worse than any of us expected. I was welcoming the thought of the ole' days of chemotherapy. One of my nurse friends called me his "little speckled trout". I am continuing a regimen of a single antibody and an antiangiogenic therapy for now and all is well.

Since re-diagnosis, I've had three different oncologists; my current doctor has been with me since 1999. I believe that we have developed a unique doctor/patient relationship. We can openly talk about medical, physical, emotional issues and especially how I am outliving that 30% life expectancy given to me so long ago and on so many occasions; we've agree it is a joint effort. I'm not sure how statistics apply to one's life, but if you're still here, you're 100% alive. I truly believe I would not be here today without his dedication and genuine concern for me as a person, not just a patient. He has true compassion for people and a passion for his vocation in life. I am honored to call him my friend. Together we have tackled all side effects; the most recurring for me has been the loss of my hair. I'm not complaining; I'm trying to convey the important message of choosing life! Do whatever it takes to make that happen. If you believe that you could never survive 10, 15 or 20 years with cancer, then you likely won't.

Realize that everyone experiences personal trauma at some point in life; how you chose to cope with it will be your life-changing moment. I have chosen to live a very productive life in the midst of cancer. The meaning of normal changes daily since this challenge began. I don't want normal to be cancer as my focus, even though it sometimes has to be part of everyday life. I choose to <u>live</u> my life first, and cancer is an afterthought.

I have set goals to visit family and friends often and travel as much as possible; not much grass grows under my feet. My doctor can only laugh and shake his head saying, "Where are you off to now?" I am fortunate to have been given opportunities to travel with family and close friends to Tahiti, Hawaii, the Bahamas, the Caribbean, from Canada to Mexico and cities from coast to coast. I have vowed not to let anything keep me from experiencing the beautiful world in which we live. One birthday, Eric gave me a skydiving trip, and my sister Trudy and I jumped out of a perfectly good airplane and loved it. Our parents thought we had lost our minds! It wasn't until I was diagnosed in 1989 that I began to truly live my life.

I am fortunate to have loving parents and stepparents, and two wonderful devoted sisters. My sister Kim had her own experience with breast cancer and sarcoma's in 1998. My sister Trudy has had numerous oncologists tell her to have her breasts removed because of our family history, she has regarded their advice. It is especially meaningful to still have my Mom who, after giving birth to me, was diagnosed with uterine/cervical cancer and given six weeks to live. She was a pioneer of chemotherapy at the National Institute of Health in Maryland in 1961. The survivorship lives on! My Dad deserves the credit for teaching me how to jump the hurdles life; always striving. My family and close friends rally around me with lots of powerful prayer and positive thoughts. I have seen seasons come and go, and with the expectation of the next, I know I will be blessed to experience the beauty of another spring and fall.

One of my biggest motivators is my beautiful daughter, Cassie. I wasn't sure I would ever see her graduate from high school; she graduated from college in the spring of 2005 and she is becoming a massage therapist. She and I share a special mother-daughter relationship; she has been the brightest light of my life. She has grown up with the possibility of losing her Mom on any given day, but I believe she has learned many vital lessons about survival. How else can you teach lessons to your children without living through them first? If I were to pass away from this life today, I know that my daughter has been given well-rounded guidance with genuine love, moral fiber, and the values I cherish. I know she has the competence and skills to make her life whole. We laugh when I tell her she's inherited a character trait of her Mom's: she is like a teabag - she'll know her strength when she's put in hot water!

Eric and I grow closer as each year passes; we continue to celebrate our years of marriage, and they keep getting better. I feel so special to have a caring and loving husband who encourages me daily to see and do the things I feel are important to me. If not for him as an integral part of my survival, I would not be here to write these words; he is the witness to my life. He shows me the depth of his love in his eyes everyday. He is the love of my life, and I want to share as many days with him as possible.

Because of cancer, I have changed my views on healthy cooking and eating. I supplement my body with the nutrients that chemotherapy kills. I enrich my mind by reading and learning about the healing capabilities that reside in our very own brains. I feed my spirit daily with meditation, music and prayer. Healing is a collaborative effort of mind – body – spirit. I am determined to heal my body.

In retrospect, my synopsis of life as a multi-year survivor of cancer is positive. I believe conventional Western medicine has progressed enormously in the last few years but still has major strides to conquer. Ideally, future generations of physicians should look beyond the realm of chemicalizing (my word) a person to death and embrace alternative therapies. I believe a key element will involve an individual targeted and genetic approach; this is happening today. Concentrating on healing and curing is more desirable than killing healthy cells while trying to target a disease. Some doctors are beginning to realize this concept and are slowly bridging the gap with complementary medicine. My hope is that this goal becomes a higher priority.

I have not been educated through a university but have attained an education more valuable than any school curriculum because of this experience. I wouldn't trade it for anything in the world. It has made me who I am today, and I am proud that I can share these experiences with newly diagnosed cancer patients. I volunteer in a patient support program and learn something new every day I'm there. I recognize the benefits of listening to someone's fears and I know that we are linked by those fears, not by cancer, but as people. If telling my stories, or trying to make someone laugh, can keep a patient from thinking about their own situation, even for a short time, then I've made a difference.

There are so many people to whom I am grateful, especially the treatment nurses; they are my extended family and guardian angels. I cannot show enough appreciation to my family, friends and countless other people that I have never met who have been praying for me for years. The experience of writing a book has been a dream for me; I have been privileged to work with three of the most inspiring and genuinely loving people I have ever known. Pam, my co-author, has been the constant source of so many positive things in my life; she will forever hold a special place in my heart. We have bonded our souls.

Our book has a significant meaning to me and by sharing it with other cancer patients; God has revealed another purpose in my life. I have been given the gift of survival and the privilege of being a messenger to those who come after me and face this storm called cancer. I am living proof that continuing to live with cancer doesn't have to make you a victim. I am not defined by it and I am not cancer Terri.   What *you do* does not define *who you are*; what defines us is how well *you rise after falling*.

Living courageously with this disease is a powerful example to people who are facing this difficult diagnosis and being able to use the knowledge from your experience is an opportunity to help others.

With the express purpose of distributing this book, I have formed a public charity called *Wings For A Cure*…and so starts another chapter in life. *Wings* has given me another focus in my life and renewed goals to pursue.

If sharing our years of survival experience can help to light the dark moments to come or calm the torrential sea of fear that can paralyze even the most courageous, it has been worth every minute of this experience, and I consider myself forever blessed to have touched another life in such a positive way.

Terri Lynn Schexnaildre Schinazi

PART I - Diagnosis

CHAPTER ONE

Hearing the News and Coping with it

The first reaction to learning you have cancer is that you "go deaf." It is hard to hear anything past that word, and the diagnosis can be overwhelming, even devastating. Although we know that cancer does not discriminate (in fact, one out of every three people in the United States will be diagnosed with it), most of us believe that it will never happen to us.

SHOCK

The shock of having cancer makes you feel numb at first. Your senses are dulled, and your thinking is muddled and confused. It is very difficult to focus on what the doctor is saying. Your mind will shut down in the same way that your body would from a physical assault. It is important to know that this is a normal response and that you will be able to ask questions after you have had time to absorb the news.

DENIAL

You may try to convince yourself that the test results were wrong and that the diagnosis is a mistake. It's normal to question the facts that you've been given, and now may be an appropriate time to request a second opinion. Review what the doctor has told you and repeat it out loud. By doing this, your mind may be able to accept what's happening. As difficult as it is, it's important to come to grips with this news as soon as you can.

FEAR

The fear that diagnosis elicits is, in large part, fear of the unknown. Some of the questions you may have are: What is going to happen? How sick will I be? Will I need surgery? Will I lose my hair? Will I die from this? You may feel as if these questions are washing over you like waves. Try to connect with those beliefs, people, routines, or any other things that help you to establish a sense of peace. Learning more about your illness and available treatments can be helpful in relieving some fears, but it is not necessary for you to learn as much as the professionals.

Terri – Being a cancer patient/volunteer has allowed me to share stories with hundreds of cancer patients over the years. Most will agree that the treatments are not as bad as the stories they've heard. Most of the horror stories you hear are misconceptions from people who have not personally experienced the treatments. It will be difficult for some, but for most, it is merely unpleasant. The side effect drugs used today will diminish or eliminate side effects completely.

Fear and uncertainty are a part of life. Try to identify your specific fears and those things you may not be able to handle, and address those issues. Meeting with a counselor can be most helpful in this process

Nancy – Fear is one of the most difficult challenges of living with a chronic illness – fear of dying, fear of losing control of your life and other fears. Let's look at fear letter by letter and break it down into ways you can deal with it: F-E-A-R.

F-Face it.   E-Examine it.   A-Ask for help.   R-Release it.

WHY ME?

Disease is a natural part of living, and no one is immune to illness or difficulty. You may feel as if you've been singled out, that you are being punished, or that you did something to deserve cancer. Don't believe it! There is no one single cause of cancer, and it's not something you bring on yourself. You can't control what's happened, but you can control how you deal with it. Don't focus on why you got cancer; focus on what you are going to do about it and how you can find purpose and meaning in the experience.

Susan - Once, before being discharged from the hospital after a particularly difficult surgery, my doctor stopped by for a visit. He told me that how the script of my life was to be written after I got home was largely up to me. I could go home, feel very sorry for myself...or, I could send the message that I didn't want pity. I decided that my goal was to feel optimistic and good about myself.

ISOLATION/LONLINESS

Susan - I remember being in the grocery store shortly after a re-diagnosis and trying to stay focused on my grocery list. I looked around and thought that no one looked like they had a care in the world. I felt like stopping people and saying, "Do you have any idea what I am going through?" I knew that these people also had problems, some worse than mine, but that wasn't how I felt. I felt isolated and alone, as if my situation were somehow different.

A sense of community is important in dealing with any event in life, particularly disease. When you are diagnosed with cancer, you feel alone. No one can walk in your shoes, but you can have someone walk alongside you. Life seems to go on around you when your world is spiraling out of control. Try to speak with someone who is going through a similar situation. Talk to other patients about their experiences, join a support group, or ask if there is someone who can call you at home to talk.

WORRY

Worrying about what may happen to you robs you of the present.

Pam – I remember as a young working adult going on a vacation and thinking on Monday, "Next Monday I'll be back at my desk." All day I would think about how few days I had left until I had to go back to work. I did that every day of the vacation and ruined the valuable time I had. After that, I realized that if I carried that way of thinking to the extreme, I would never enjoy anything because everything eventually ends. I decided to relish each moment because since all things end, they are more precious. It's also like a child to say that because a game will eventually end, I might as well not play. On the contrary, because it will end, we need to give it our best effort.

You can take on all kinds of problems that may never happen, and in so doing, you take on additional stress and most importantly, you miss the joy of the moment.

Nancy – I knew a woman who was having a very difficult time moving on with her life. For months she had allowed cancer to steal her joy and consume her life. I had the opportunity to share some things with her that had helped me on my cancer journey, and she began to focus less on cancer and more on living. About two months later she was killed in a car wreck. When I heard the news, I thought how sad it was that she had spent so many months imprisoned by cancer instead of making memories and enjoying life.

The past is over, and you can't change it; the future is unknowable, and no amount of wishing will make it predictable; however, you do have the present, and it is your most valuable currency. Spend it wisely. Take on only the problems you face at the moment. Phrases like, "Don't borrow trouble," and, "Cross that bridge when you come to it," are clichés because so many people have realized the truth of them in their own lives. Life is happening while you are worrying.

Susan – During a particularly difficult time, I scheduled a 15-minute worry period into my day. I used this period of time each day to deal with all the "what if's," then I would try to put them away until my worry time the next day. If your mind occasionally takes you to the land of "what if" (What if I get another tumor? What if this treatment doesn't work? What if they find something else during surgery?), be assured that this is natural. Try to make a conscious effort to limit your worry time. As you wait for test results, diagnoses, treatments and appointments, remember that you are living now. Even among the challenges of life, there are countless wonderful and amazing things to see and do in each moment if we look for them.

ANGER

There are many aspects of a cancer diagnosis that may trigger feelings of anger: loss of control, a change in lifestyle, low energy levels, hair loss, etc. It is normal to be angry when your life has been turned upside down and your routines are disrupted. Remember that anger is neither right nor wrong; it's simply an emotion that can range from slight irritation to absolute fury. Don't feel guilty about being angry, but do acknowledge it so that you can move on beyond it. If you don't find an outlet to express your anger, you can easily turn it inward and become depressed. For some patients, however, anger can be an important component of survival because it gives them the will and determination to live. Expressing your anger can be healthy, but it is important to find productive ways to do so and not let it consume and control your life. When you feel angry, try to find appropriate outlets to help relieve the frustrations you may be feeling.

Things that might help:

- Distract yourself with a movie or shopping.
- Discuss your feelings with a friend.

- Try to resolve issues; for example, being kept waiting for a medical appointment can cause anger and frustration, but seething about it won't help solve the problem. It is much more productive to discuss this with your medical team to find ways to resolve it in the future.

- Discuss your anger with a counselor.

It is also common for friends and family to experience the same feelings of anger and frustration. While your anger should be directed toward the disease, it can sometimes be misdirected to the people around you. Make agreements with others to be open and honest about how you are feeling. This will help to eliminate additional stress for everyone concerned.

As we were writing this book, three of us were facing new challenges and taking new treatments. We realized that although we didn't choose this direction for our lives, we could control how we handled what happened to us. We focused on the fact that we can control our attitudes, and we can direct our anger in positive directions.

DEPRESSION

Life can present challenges and stresses during every phase, even when you are well. When the stress of cancer is added, you can easily become depressed. Don't be embarrassed about your feelings; acknowledge them and monitor them just as you would your physical symptoms.

Be aware of these marked changes in your routine:

- Feeling depressed most of the day, nearly every day

- Having trouble sleeping, or spending most of your day in bed
- Loss of interest in doing the things that usually bring you pleasure
- Loss of appetite
- or constant eating
- Loss of concentration or inability to make decisions.

Any of these symptoms can be the result of medications or drug interactions, or they can be signs of depression.

Susan - I experienced short periods of several of these symptoms. Sometimes I would get into bed feeling exhausted, but I would be unable to turn my mind off so that I could sleep. At other times, I felt as if my motor were running in high gear. On occasion, I would flit from task to task unable to stay focused on any one thing long enough to get it completed.

Be careful not to fall into the smiling-depressed disorder, which is smiling through your pain or suffering, trying not to burden those around you and masking what you really feel. Talk to your physician about how you feel emotionally. It is equally important for your doctor to know that you are having trouble getting out of bed because you feel depressed as to know that you are in bed due to nausea. Both situations can be helped with medication. Remember not to lose sight of what is good in your life. Accept the love and support of those who care about you and the professional expertise of your medical caregivers. (see also PART IV, Depression.)

WHAT NOW?

Try not to add to your stress by thinking you absolutely have to understand your diagnosis, the terminology being used or the treatment options being proposed. This experience will be an ongoing education for you and your family. Allow yourself some time to absorb the news. Your physician or a staff member should be available to review all information and answer your questions over the course of the next few days, weeks, or months. Being a cancer patient is one of life's greatest challenges. As simplistic as it sounds, try to take it one step at a time. Sometimes the anticipation of what a procedure or treatment will be like is worse than the reality. Once you have seen your doctors, obtained a second or third opinion and completed your research, you may feel overwhelmed with the decisions you have to make. (see also CHAPTER THREE – Second Opinions.) This is one of the most challenging parts of dealing with cancer. Prepared with your information, go into a quiet room alone, turn off the phone, relax and let your intuition be your guide; listen to your inner voice. If you are unsure about what you need to do, take a sheet of paper and draw a line down the middle, with positives on one side and negatives on the other. All cancer treatments are a balance between risks and side effects. Writing it on paper will enable you to see more clearly what your options are. If you still need additional information, you may want to talk to your doctor. When you have made the decision, don't look back and say, "I wish I had done..." You made the best choice you could based on the information you had at the time. Don't try to second-guess yourself or let others cause you to doubt your decisions. Move ahead with confidence.

TWO IMPORTANT ASPECTS FOR EMOTIONAL WELL BEING

Attitude

A positive attitude does have a powerful effect on your immune system, and it can make life more enjoyable for you and those around you. Having a positive attitude doesn't mean denial; it means that you face the situation and try to look for the good in it. Believing that life is good and truly taking enjoyment in it can help to offset the stress related to cancer treatment. After all, your goal is to complete your treatments so you can move on to a fulfilling life. Having a good attitude can make a big difference in how you deal with the experience of your illness, but it doesn't mean that you can avoid being worried or even scared some of the time

Nancy - Most importantly, you should remember that cancer is a six-letter word, and the first three letters of that word spell can. You CAN do this!

Take it one day at a time; learn from the experiences of those who have gone before you, and be assured that you do not have to go through this alone.

Humor

Most people would think there isn't anything funny about having cancer, but if you let it rob you of the ability to laugh you have given up a great healing resource. Laughter may be the most underrated means of healing. At this time in your life when you feel that there isn't much to laugh about, humor will help to keep you from falling into depression. Most survivors will agree that there are many humorous moments in the course of your cancer journey. Part of being a patient involves being prodded, poked, exposed, photographed, and embarrassed, etc. Make the best of it and choose to enjoy the moments of laughter.

Nancy – I am a great believer in the importance of hugs. I regularly dispense hugs, and I like receiving them in return. Physicians sometimes have trouble reciprocating. One doctor in particular was very reserved. I explained my "hug therapy" policy and proceeded to give him a little hug at the start of each visit. One day he decided that he was also ready to dispense a hug; I was sitting on the examining table dressed in my formal gown. As he crossed the room and reached out to give me a hug, his foot hit the lever that controls the examining table, and up went the table causing him to stumble and fall on top of me. I think that probably set him back in his progress with "hug therapy," but it certainly provided a laugh for the day and a good feeling that he had crossed the hug threshold.

Use laughter to heal; it can reduce blood pressure, release endorphins and make you look and feel better. It's contagious and is something you can share with other people. Surround yourself with happy people and people who make you laugh; their joy will lighten your spirit when you need it the most. Watch funny movies, read humorous books, and try to keep some fun in your life. Remember that life is much too important to be taken seriously.

Susan - I particularly recall one cancer patient losing her hair while having a bone marrow transplant. She purchased a tiara, and each day when she reported to the bone marrow transplant clinic for treatment, she placed the tiara on her bald head and called herself the "Princess of Chemo."

You have only so much control at this time in your life, and one thing you can control is your focus. Focusing on what is good tends to make it a little easier to smile even during the difficult times.

Terri – Of the 12 or so nurses at my treatment clinic, there is one male nurse in the hen house. It is amazing to watch the interaction between the other nurses and him, but even more so with the patients. He brings laughter into the clinic as often as possible and wins the hearts of patients with his unique sense of humor and infectious giggle. He never misses a chance to reel me in to a practical joke or fictitious story. Some of the other nurses will join in the fun and on many occasions the roar of laughter can be heard throughout the halls. Having laughter in a treatment room is a healing experience to behold.

CHAPTER TWO
Telling Family and Friends

When you learn you have cancer, you will find that family and friends will become a very important part of healing. But how do you break the news? When you get new information, you have to assimilate it yourself before you can tell others. You will know intuitively when it is the right time. Try to find a trusted and calm family member or friend with whom you can share so that you are not carrying this burden alone. How you handle your news and how you share it with others will determine their attitudes about your situation. If you are open and honest and let them know that you feel comfortable talking about your diagnosis, then they will not fear that they might say something to upset you. It is difficult for some people to face the fact that someone they love has cancer. Some people may avoid you. Try not to be hurt or offended - it doesn't mean they love you less; it just means that they have a difficult time expressing themselves about your situation. Encourage them to ask questions and talk with you. Tell your family when new information becomes available so they won't feel as though you are keeping something from them. After all, they are part of your healing team, and they need to know your condition in order to help you.

Susan - Cancer seems to give people permission to tell you how much they love you. It is amazing how people will say, "I love you" to a cancer patient, when before they wouldn't have felt free to express that. Take advantage of this opportunity to absorb all the love others have for you.

It is not necessary to inform everyone about your illness immediately. Tell people when you feel comfortable sharing the news with them. One word of caution: it is preferable that those close to you hear the news directly from you or someone you choose, rather than getting the news secondhand. This will help to dispel incorrect information and unnecessary confusion about your health. Well-meaning friends may have many cancer stories for you. Savor the encouraging ones, and try to dismiss the "everything went wrong" variety.

Telling your Children

When considering how your cancer affects the lives of your children, you need to take into account many factors, among them: ✔ the ages of your children ✔ whether or not you, the patient, are the primary parent ✔ how incapacitated you may be following surgery or during treatment ✔ if you will be separated from your children during this time. Just as you may be feeling uncertain about how you will deal with all of this, you can't be sure exactly how your children will respond. However, be assured that for the most part, children are amazingly resilient. Although they will take their cues from you and other caregivers, that does not mean that you must "put on a happy face" all of the time. Children are often better able to show their concerns if we express some of ours in a way appropriate to their age and ability to understand.

Susan – My eleven-year-old daughter wisely told me that it would be easier for her to cry if I would let her see me cry once in a while.

It is important for your children to learn the news of your cancer directly from you. Exactly what you tell them will be determined by their ages. Choose a time and place where you will have privacy with no interruptions. It is helpful to have your spouse or another family member present. Tell them the basic information: that you have an illness called cancer, where it is located in your body and what treatment you will be having. Then encourage their questions, and answer them honestly in a simple and direct manner. Being honest with them is better than allowing them to think the worst. Be sure to tell younger children that they cannot get cancer from you and that they have not done anything to cause you to get cancer. Don't be surprised or offended if younger children listen to the news, ask a question or two, and then inquire if they can go play. Bring the subject up again at various times so they can become comfortable with the information and feel at ease talking to you about it. Keep their daily routine as regular as possible. If certain activities need to be adjusted, give them as much warning as you can. Children are quite adaptable, but they will adjust more easily to this change if a sense of structure is maintained. During the course of your treatments it is appropriate for everyone to have occasional treats. A trip for an ice cream sundae "just because" can be therapeutic for all involved. However, dispensing gifts or fulfilling unusual requests is not normal and can actually be hard for a child to understand. It is important that children realize that an adult is still supervising everyday events. Now more than ever, they need the safety net of knowing that someone is watching out for them. If you are separated from your children, communicate through phone calls, e-mail, notes, audio or videotapes. You may want to record bedtime stories, which can be played in your absence. Be sure that they understand when and why you will be away. If you are going to lose your hair or have body markings during radiation treatment, make certain they know what's going to happen to you and understand it. Doing things to help your children feel more comfortable with your illness may also allow you to be more at ease with some of the side effects of your cancer and its treatment. (For example, maybe you can get matching hats or caps when you lose your hair.) Most importantly, continue to let your children know that you love them, and dispense lots of hugs and kisses. Not only is that essential for their well-being, but getting the return of hugs and kisses will allow you to receive some of the best therapy there is!

Your Child With Cancer

If it is your child who has cancer, you should take him/her to a children's cancer center, if possible. Cancer can be one of the most frightening diseases that a child can face. The good news is that almost 80% of children with cancer can be cured with early detection and treatment. Children's cancer centers are best equipped to deal with the special needs that a child's cancer involves. See the Resource section in this book.

PART II - Essentials

CHAPTER THREE

Being a Cancer Patient

The amount of information you may want about your illness and treatment may vary. Some patients prefer to be very well-informed, while others want to play a less active role in the decision-making. Neither way is right or wrong; the important thing is to do what is best for you. Initially, the doctor may explain some basic facts about the type of cancer you have and discuss additional diagnostic tests and options for courses of treatment. It is important that you understand the implications of your particular medical situation and the goal of the treatment plan your medical team is suggesting. Focusing on the facts can be challenging at this particular time. Try to understand what you are being told, and realize that it may be difficult to stay focused.

COMMUNICATING WITH YOUR DOCTOR

Take special care to develop a good working relationship with your doctor since you are partners in your treatment.

- Select a physician who regularly treats the type of cancer you have. If the doctor is in private practice, learn what hospital(s) s/he is affiliated with and if s/he participates in research programs or clinical trials.

- You should be able to ask your doctor questions with ease, and if you are not comfortable with that, then you need to find another doctor.

- Be prepared for your visits with your doctor. You may have several doctors involved in your care depending upon the treatment plan, so remember your notepad of questions, and write down the answers. Again, always let him/her know if you will be taping the conversation.

- Don't pretend to understand what has been said if you don't. Continue to ask questions until it is clear. Repeating what you have heard enables the doctor to know whether you understood correctly, and to clarify any point that you may have misunderstood.

- If you have a question that the doctor may need time to evaluate, try to submit the question prior to your visit. Ask your doctor which is the best way to communicate with him/her and whether s/he responds to e-mail.

- You should inform your doctor of any emotional or psychological issues or unusual sources of stress in your life.

- Inform your doctor of anything that may affect your medical care, including herbal and dietary supplements, vitamins, minerals, and over-the-counter medications that you may be taking. Certain vitamins or supplements can interfere with the effectiveness of the treatment.

Some patients allow their physicians to make all the decisions about their treatment. If this is your choice, then you must clearly communicate it to your doctor. Other patients find it empowering to learn all they can about their illness from the very beginning. If you decide at some point that you want more information about treatment options, let your healthcare team know that you want to be more involved in making those decisions. How often you see your doctor(s) will be determined by your treatment plan. Between treatment appointments, try to go about your normal routine as much as possible. Your medical team will discuss common side effects that might occur as a result of your treatment (see PART IV, Side Effects). It is important to contact your doctor immediately if you should experience any unexpected side effects. Do not assume it is too insignificant to let him/her know about the problem.

WHEN YOU HAVE SEVERAL DOCTORS

Since more than one doctor may see you in the course of your treatment, you may wonder when and with whom you should interact. You will be consulting with an oncologist, a doctor who specializes in the treatment of cancer. Three types of oncologists that you may have to meet with are:

- Surgical oncologists - specialize in the surgical removal of the cancer
- Radiation oncologists - specialize in treating the cancer with radiation
- Medical oncologists - specialize in treating the cancer with drugs.

In the course of making your decision about treatment, you may see one or a combination of all three oncologists; when the treatment protocol is chosen, one or more of these oncologists may be involved in treating your cancer. Be sure to learn the following things:

- The doctor who is in charge of directing your treatment
- How to contact each of your attending physicians
- If all files and records pertaining to each phase of your treatment are being sent to each doctor
- The appropriate person to contact regarding specific questions or concerns.

You are likely to have a favorite doctor with whom you can best communicate. Even if you are at a phase in your treatment when you are not seeing that doctor regularly, let him/her know that you would like to stay in touch and ask the best way to accomplish this. You need to realize that the physician you prefer may not be in charge of your current treatment and may need to defer to the doctor who is.

SECOND OPINIONS

It is important to obtain good medical advice and get a second and possibly a third opinion, preferably from a National Cancer Institute (NCI) designated comprehensive cancer center. Don't let anyone rush you into making a decision. Some patients don't seek a second opinion because it is too inconvenient or they are afraid they will insult the first doctor with whom they consulted. Remember that you don't get a second chance to do it right, so you want to make sure that you have made the best decision before you move forward with treatment, surgery or radiation. You will find a list of books, phone numbers, and websites in the

Resource section of this book that will help guide you through the decision-making process.

You can self-refer to any comprehensive cancer center or other facility. Through the NCI service (1-800-4-CANCER) you can learn the name and location of oncologists specializing in the type of cancer you have. Independently arranging for another opinion provides you the assurance that you have received an unbiased opinion. It is important that you make this visit in person and take your pathology slides and all of your medical records and scans or x-rays with you. *Note: Because of HIPAA, the new federal regulations designed to protect your privacy as a patient, hospitals and doctors are unable to access your medical records without your consent. Consider joining MedicAlert® so that your personal medical information is readily available in a medial emergency.*

Most insurance companies will pay for a second opinion, but you should check with your insurance provider for specifics of your plan. If they will not pay for it, consider paying for it yourself. Do everything you can to get the best advice possible.

HOW TO LET OTHERS HELP YOU

Think about how your family members and friends can support you and how they can help you to cope. Assigning responsibilities to loved ones can be very helpful and also allow them to feel they have a significant role in your care.

- **Visits to the doctor** – Have someone help you organize your questions prior to visits or phone conversations to your doctor. You may want to ask a family member or friend to accompany you to appointments to take notes.

- **Treatments** – You may want to ask a friend to go with you when you have your radiation or chemotherapy treatments. This gives you an opportunity to visit with each other throughout the day. Ask someone to coordinate a rotating schedule and invite other friends to drive you to the clinic for your treatment. For example, if you are having daily radiation treatments, perhaps five people would consider taking you – one for each day of the week. It's helpful to have a backup who can substitute if one of the "regulars" has a conflict. Some people schedule a friend per week, especially if they are from out of town and are staying in a hotel.

- **Preparing meals** – If neighbors or a church or temple group are planning to bring meals to you, ask them to arrange for someone to coordinate the schedule. Let the person handling the arrangements know if there are dietary restrictions so they can prepare meals accordingly. Having dinner brought each night usually results in a vast quantity of leftovers. Every other night often works better and makes the generosity of others last longer. Friends could also bring casseroles, which can be frozen for later use.

- **Children** – The amount of help you need will depend upon the ages of the children. To give you some quiet time, friends and family can take your children out to dinner, invite them over to play with their children, or they can baby-sit while you go out for a break. They can also take them to school, pick them up, and give them rides to after-school activities. The children may need help with homework while you are not feeling up to par, so ask a friend to lend a hand.

- **Errands/ Shopping/ Mail/Personal** – If you need groceries, clothes, household items or gifts for others, ask someone to do your shopping or run other errands for you. You could have a neighbor get mail, buy stamps, write notes or pick up prescriptions. Have a family member or close friend drive you to personal appointments for manicures, pedicures or other beauty treatments.

- **Phone calls** – You can use an answering machine to screen your calls. If you receive lots of calls, you may want to record a message with updates on your condition or other contact information. Doing this allows you to return calls when it is convenient for you. Don't feel obligated to answer the phone when you are not feeling well.

- **Visits from friends** – People who stop by without calling first mean well, but you may not feel like having visitors. Don't feel that you have to entertain on someone else's schedule. You may want to leave a note on the door with a pad and pencil. You can explain that you don't feel like having visitors at the present, and ask them to leave a note so you will know they were there. Let your friends know if you would like to have visitors when you are in the hospital or if you need someone to stay with you at any time.

- **E-mail Updates** – A great way to communicate your current condition with family and friends is to send an e-mail newsletter. This is very helpful to keep everyone informed, especially if you don't feel well enough to keep repeating your medical stories. There are also many e-mail services that offer free websites that you can use to update how you are feeling and give other medical information when someone wants to check up on you.

- **Housecleaning/Yard Work** – Since you may need regular help with your housecleaning, friends can assist you, or a group of them can pool their resources and hire someone to clean. If laundry becomes overwhelming, ask someone to wash, dry and fold the clothes (and then have a family member put them away). Friends can mow the lawn, take care of your plants or help with other yard work.

- **Pet Care** – If you have a pet, you might need help caring for it when you feel fatigued. Consider asking a friend to walk your dog, take the pet to the vet or just visit with you and play with the pet when it needs some exercise or attention.

- **Flowers/Cards/Magazines/Books/Tapes** – Let friends know when you receive flowers and cards that you appreciate it. Also, let them know what kind of books you like to read and what music you like. Often, when you are having treatment, you may not feel like reading, or you may find that your concentration isn't as focused, so books on tape work well.

- **Bills** – You can request help in managing your accounting and paying your bills if necessary. (It is very convenient to set up bill paying online.)

- **Social Activities/Entertainment** – How you feel will vary from day-to-day. You may have a compromised immune system, which prevents you from being in crowds, or you might not feel up to being sociable. You can ask friends to include you anyway, but to understand if you need to decline because you don't have the energy. If you feel up to it, ask a friend to join you for a movie, take you for a ride, or join you for a luncheon date.

- **Spouse Night Out** – Encourage your spouse to take advantage of some much-needed personal time; you can use this opportunity to invite friends to visit you.

- **Driving** – Operating a vehicle depends on the type, amount and potency of the medication you will be taking. If you are taking something that will impair your senses, don't drive. In the initial stages of chemotherapy, several drugs are given to eliminate the possibility of an adverse reaction. It is recommended that you have a ride home after your chemo treatments in the event you have a drug reaction. After a few treatments with no adverse reactions, you may be able to discontinue any additional medication and resume driving. However, you must first get approval from your doctor if you have been restricted from driving.

You may find that friends and family will begin to hover around you, so you should give them guidance about how much freedom you want while you recuperate. Lovingly let them know how and when they can help. Explain to your friends and family that you may need some time alone.

The people closest to you will want to be there for you, but they may feel helpless because they don't know what to do. Be honest, and tell them your needs. Frequently well-intentioned friends and family will suggest books, articles, web sites or tapes that they think would be helpful; this advice can be overwhelming. Follow your intuition, and use only those resources that suit your needs.

Caregivers

Pam – As a caregiver, remember the person who has cancer is still the same person as before, only one with a problem. Perhaps the greatest gift we can give our friends is to treat them normally. Offer help, but don't make them feel different. (After all, we all have problems, and we all get sick.) Let them enjoy the good times and share troubles just as you always do. Including them in all aspects of life and allowing them to participate as fully as possible, will let them know that you realize we are all connected and that they are not alone. Being connected and loving is what we are all called to be to each other.

KEEPING A MEDICAL JOURNAL

A medical journal is a good way to keep a record of many things, including the following: ✔ your medications ✔ treatments and your reactions to them ✔ appointments ✔ diagnostic test results ✔ blood work ✔ lab results. A spiral notebook, with dividers for each category, is very useful for this type of record keeping. You should take your medical journal with you to all appointments so you will have the pertinent information you need to discuss with your doctor. Reviewing this journal can help you to identify recurrent physical patterns or symptoms that you are experiencing. It is also very useful to take your journal, or a simplified medical history sheet, with you when you travel in the event you get sick or have a medical emergency.

CHAPTER FOUR

Practical Concerns

APPOINTMENTS

Appointments are a part of life during any treatment protocol. Recognize that the tests may take all day, so be prepared to wait. Sometimes things go smoothly when you arrive for an appointment or test, but it is best to be prepared for any delay. Things to remember for appointments:

- Medications you may need to take while waiting

- A list of your current medications (remember to note the dosage and frequency)

- Current insurance information, Medicare, or Medicaid cards

- Allergy information (drugs you have had reactions to)

- A written list of questions for your doctor

- A small voice recorder to replay information (make sure to ask permission to use the recorder during your appointment) or to use to listen to music while you are waiting or receiving your treatment

- A snack, something to read, a word puzzle, a small craft project or writing paper.

Many treatment facilities have resource centers, which can be a great source of information, especially while you are waiting. Ask if the treatment center offers a wig/turban loan program and if they have self-help groups, support group meetings, and if counselors are available.

Note: It is recommended that you have any necessary dental work completed before you make your appointment for your treatments.

RECORD KEEPING

Due to the strict specifications of HIPAA, the new federal regulations designed to protect your privacy as a patient, hospitals and doctors are unable to access your medical records without your consent. Always carry with you a list of important medical information such as drug allergies, current medications indicating dosage and frequency, previous surgeries or illnesses, and the name and phone numbers of your current and previous doctors.

Your medical records (i.e., insurance, tests results, invoices, etc.) are very important documents and should be managed with care. The information in your records is used to help process your appointment more efficiently. Your organized records can also be used to answer important insurance questions and can be invaluable if you decide to visit another medical center for a second opinion. It may be helpful to keep records in a file drawer or an accordion file folder. Some important things to remember:

- Make yourself a copy of any files you have sent to another facility.

- When you talk to anyone regarding your insurance or benefits, write down the date, time, the person's name and key points of the conversation.

- If you are told in person or by phone about a decision to correct a billing error, be sure to ask for a written confirmation of the correction.

- Request itemized copies of bills for hospitalization and outpatient treatments.

- Ask if your treatment facility has a policy of purging films, slides or x-rays after so many years; if that is the case, it is important that you ask for them to be sent to you instead. Keep track of where your films and slides are kept.

- Keep a record of all medical expenses such as parking, hotels, travel (mileage), etc., - some of these may be tax deductible. The IRS provides a list of deductible expenses.

- Maintain a separate file for each year of your care.

- Do not pay any bill without checking it for accuracy.

MEDICAL DIRECTIVES

Once you have decided on your treatment protocol, you should get your advanced medical directives in order. Make sure you have a current will, and write down or tell someone your final arrangement details. It is not pessimistic to deal with these matters, but practical and realistic to take care of difficult things before they happen. It is a fact that everyone dies eventually, and making the decisions about your death beforehand will make it easier for the people who love you to handle your personal business. Other advanced directives you should consider are a living will, a healthcare power of attorney, a general durable power of attorney, and a Do-Not-Resuscitate (DNR).

A *living will* is a written document that states your desired medical care should you become terminally ill or in a permanent vegetative state. It is also known as a declaration of desire for a natural death. You should be specific about what medical procedures you want provided or withheld and for what duration. This document must be notarized and signed by two witnesses.

A *healthcare power of attorney* is a legal document in which you name a person to make medical decisions for you if you become unable to make them for yourself. You should state what medical treatments you would or would not want performed, and you name an adult you trust to be your healthcare agent. This document must be notarized and signed by two witnesses. A *general durable power of attorney* is a document in which you name a person to handle your financial affairs in the event that your doctor states you have become medically incapacitated. It must be notarized and signed by two witnesses. A *Do-Not-Resuscitate (DNR)* order is an advanced directive to medical professionals not to attempt emergency CPR if your breathing or heartbeat stops. A DNR directive can be included in your living will or can be stated directly to your physician. You or your healthcare agent can remove the DNR by telling your doctor, nurses, or others of your decision. See website listings in the Resource sections for more information.

FINANCIAL CONSIDERATIONS

Cancer is an expensive illness. You and your family may be troubled about your finances. Besides hospital bills and medications, cancer treatment includes many expenses that insurance doesn't pay. Ask to talk with a hospital social worker for help in accessing financial aid. See also our Resources section for excellent sources in getting financial help when you need it.

PART III

Understanding Procedures

CHAPTER FIVE

How to Prepare For Tests

Your physician will routinely schedule medical tests in the course of monitoring your treatment and investigating your symptoms. You might feel uneasy or frightened about undergoing an unfamiliar procedure, but knowing how to prepare and what to expect can help you to be comfortable and make the tests go more smoothly. Again, recognize that the tests may take all day, so be prepared to wait. Try not to borrow trouble. Sometimes when people know they are going to be tested, they begin to experience symptoms they didn't notice until then (the power of suggestion). Remember that it's possible to have a normal headache or stomachache even when you have cancer. As a cancer patient, you must always be mindful of the messages your body sends you, but you must take the circumstances into consideration.

- Clothing Guideline - To avoid wearing those skimpy gowns or having to change your clothes, you should wear clothing that has no metal in it. Jogging suits with plastic zippers or pants with elastic in the waist work well. You may want to wear a sports bra with no metal, or simply remove your bra prior to the procedure if that is the only article of clothing with metal. During the cooler months, try wearing sweat suits or jogging suits. In the warmer months, scrubs are a comfortable choice.

- Pregnancy – Be sure to inform the nurse or technician if you are pregnant or if there is a possibility that you could be pregnant.

- Relaxation Techniques – Learn and use a few simple relaxation techniques to help you avoid test anxiety and discomfort. Some simple breathing exercises can help you to relax and minimize apprehension (see CHAPTER TEN – Breathwork and Meditation). If you are still uneasy, you can ask the technician to request a mild sedative for you from your doctor.

CHAPTER SIX

Common Types of Tests

BIOPSY

When a suspicious lump has been discovered, or if x-rays reveal an abnormal area, your doctor may choose to take a biopsy (tissue sample) to be examined under a microscope. The biopsy will reveal whether the tissue is cancerous. One type of biopsy may be done with a needle; this is called a fine needle aspiration biopsy. The needle is inserted directly into the lump (tumor or cyst) or affected area to draw out cells into a syringe to determine if the lump is cancerous. In a core needle biopsy a special needle is used to obtain small cylinders of tissue for diagnostic evaluation. An ultrasound machine may also be used to direct the needle into the mass for accuracy. An excisional biopsy, also called a lumpectomy, is the surgical removal of an entire mass and possibly some of the surrounding tissue. An incisional biopsy is one in which the surgeon cuts into the tumor and removes part or all of it. You doctor will determine the anesthesia to be used during the biopsy procedure. See Surgery, this chapter.

BLOODWORK

Your blood counts will be measured prior to your treatment to determine if they are at a safe level. Your blood is a vital part of the messaging system of your body. It is a river that carries oxygen from your lungs to every cell in your body, glucose from your digestive system to all your cells for energy, and waste products from cells to organs for elimination. Doctors use information found in your blood to gauge the internal health of your body, and to diagnose and manage disease. Although blood appears to be just a red liquid, it is actually composed of a pale, yellow liquid called plasma and billions of cells. In addition to cells, plasma contains other substances such as chemicals, enzymes, minerals, vitamins and hormones. Most of your blood cells are red, which give blood its color, and they carry oxygen. They are composed primarily of a substance rich in iron, called hemoglobin. Your white blood cells help your body to fight infection, and your platelets enable your blood to clot, thereby stopping bleeding. Blood is made in spongy tissue in the middle of the bone, called bone marrow. Cells divide very quickly in bone marrow, and since chemotherapy affects quickly dividing cells (like cancer cells) it will affect your bone marrow. Because your blood cells won't have been replaced at the normal rate, there won't be as many cells, and your counts will be low. Your dosage may be reduced or your treatment postponed. Your doctor may prescribe medications to help bring up the counts. When a therapy is delayed because of low counts, it does not mean that the cancer will grow out of control.

Blood Counts

A blood count is the measurement of the number of blood cells a person has in his/her circulation as shown in a laboratory sample of blood. Blood cells divide rapidly; since chemotherapy targets rapidly dividing cells (like cancer), it also affects blood cells.

When you are having chemotherapy, your blood cell production is suppressed. Because of low blood counts, you may feel tired and listless, and you might be subject to more infections and have an increased risk of bleeding easily.

- When your red blood counts are low (anemia), you may experience fatigue, breathing difficulty, dizziness, feeling cold or a rapid heartbeat.

- When you have a low white blood count, you may develop a fever or an infection.

- When you have a low platelet count, you can bruise more easily, bleed more easily, and/or have nosebleeds.

If this occurs, your doctor may prescribe various bone marrow stimulants to help produce more blood cells. A complete blood count, called a CBC, is a very common test, and your doctor will order it on a regular basis. It identifies the types, amounts and characteristics of your blood cells.

What a CBC Measures

- RBC (red blood cells) (Also called erythrocytes) - Carry oxygen and remove waste. Measured in millions per cubic millimeter of blood (mil/mm).

- HGB (hemoglobin)-Protein part of red blood cell. Measured in terms of weight.

- HCT (hematocrit)- Percentage of blood made of red cells. Measured in percentage.

- Platelets - (Also called thrombocytes) Cells that help stop bleeding by clotting. Measured as platelets in one-millionth of a liter (microliter - μL).

- WBC (white blood cells) - (Also called leukocytes) Help the body fight infection. Measured in thousands per cubic milliliter (K/mm).

- Differential ABC (automated blood count) - Measures five specific types of white blood cells. Measured as a percentage of all white blood cells.

- Neutrophils - Cells that fight against infection.

- Lymphocytes (B and T cells) - Create antibodies, attack foreign invaders.

- Monocytes - Ingest foreign material.

- Eosinophils - Destroy parasites, respond to allergic reactions.

- Basophils - Play a major role in inflammation.

Blood Chemistry

Another type of test your doctor may order is a blood chemistry, which analyzes the plasma (serum), the liquid portion of your blood in which the cells and platelets travel. A blood chemistry profile will include values for substances such as electrolytes (like sodium {Na} or potassium {K}), liver enzymes (like alkaline phosphatase, bilirubin), kidney function tests (like blood urea nitrogen {BUN} creatinine), protein, lipids (cholesterol), thyroid function tests, glucose, and iron. These tests, along with others, are used to help track the progression of your disease and help the doctor to make decisions about your treatment. If you need more details, you may want to have a health care professional explain what the numbers mean. You can also look up information in medical reference manuals, go to the library or search the internet.

BONE SCAN

Bone scans are used to determine if cancer has spread to the bones. A bone scan is commonly used in patients with breast, prostate or lung cancers, as well as lymphoma. It can detect lesions three to six months before they appear on an X-ray, making it valuable in evaluating bone pain.

Things to know when going for your bone scan:

- Follow clothing guidelines in CHAPTER FIVE, How to Prepare For Tests.

- When you arrive, you will be asked for your weight, and a low-dose radioactive substance will be prepared for you. The technician will inject that substance into a vein. If you have poor veins, you should start exercising your veins by squeezing a rubber ball before you arrive and several days prior to the scan. You can build the muscles around your veins, which gives them more support and makes them easier to access. If you have veins that are difficult to access, inform the technician. Share with your nurse any helpful hints to help access your best veins.

- Following the injection, there is a waiting period of two hours. You should drink as much fluid as you can (at least two large glasses). The radioactive substance that is injected will attach to the bone cells, and any excess will flush out through the kidneys and bladder. Your goal is to drink fluid to accelerate that process.

- You can bring a CD or tape player or an iPod so that you can listen to relaxing music while you are having your scan.

- You should avoid being in close contact with pregnant women for 24 hours after radioactive injection.

The scanning procedure is simple and comfortable because you are lying on a table with the scanner above you. It is very close to your body, and you must lie very still. Results of the scan will be sent to your doctor, and the doctor will discuss them with you by phone or a visit in the office.

CAT OR CT SCAN

A CAT or CT scan (computed axial tomography) is a machine that uses advanced x-rays of the same part of the body from different angles. The image results are detailed cross-sections of your internal organs. You may be asked to drink a contrast liquid. There are choices of liquid contrast; be sure to ask the nurse what they are and which would be best for you. Depending on the area being scanned, you may be told not to eat prior to your test. You may also receive IV contrast during the scan; be sure to let the technician or nurse know if you've previously had an allergic reaction to iodine. When receiving the contrast "push" you will feel a warm flush throughout your body- this is not an allergic reaction; it is an expected side effect from the contrast. During the scan, you will be asked to hold your breath in short intervals so the pictures are clear. The scan takes approximately 15-30 minutes and is painless.

Things to know when going for your CAT scan:

- Follow clothing guidelines in CHAPTER FIVE, How to Prepare For Tests.

- Arrive early to complete necessary paperwork.

- To prevent upset stomach, avoid solid foods for four hours prior to the scan.

- If your doctor orders contrast, you should drink it continuously an hour and a half before the scan.

- A port cannot be used for the injected contrast; an IV must be started.

- If you are a diabetic, discontinue metformin before the scan.

CHEST X-RAY

A chest x-ray is a simple, relatively inexpensive test used to diagnose cancer, follow the progress of a disease, respond to treatment or evaluate catheter placement. X-ray images of bone, soft tissue and air can be seen easily. It can also be used as a screening tool, then followed up with a more definitive scan.

Things to know when going for your chest x-ray:

- Follow clothing guidelines in CHAPTER FIVE, How to Prepare For Tests.

- Remove all metal jewelry.

MRI

MRI (magnetic resonance imaging) is a technique that uses magnetism, radio waves and a computer to produce images of the body (not x-rays). You will be placed in a cylinder-shaped scanner that is surrounded by a magnet. The MRI doesn't hurt and has no known side effects. The test time varies based on the area being scanned. For example, a full-body scan takes much longer than a head scan.

Things to know when going for your MRI:

- Follow clothing guidelines in CHAPTER FIVE, How to Prepare For Tests.

- Remove jewelry and any metal objects.

- When you arrive for the MRI, you will be asked to complete a form to answer several questions. Since the MRI uses magnets and radio waves, you cannot take anything metal into the room with you, so you will be asked to put all of your personal belongings in a lock box until you have completed the MRI. A family member may accompany you into the room, and if one does, must also complete a form and leave his/her belongings in a lock box.

- Since any metal can distort the images obtained by the scanner, let the technician know before the exam if you have any artificial joints, bone plates or metal prosthetic implants.

- Toward the end of your scan, you may need an IV with contrast (different from a CAT scan contrast) to get better pictures. If you have poor veins and have a port, it may be used for injecting the contrast.

- Since you lie in a metal tube during the scan, you might feel "closed in" or claustrophobic. Feel free to ask the nurse for a mild sedative. Remember, deep breathing is always helpful for relaxing your body. (see Breathwork, CHAPTER TEN.)

- An MRI makes loud repetitive clicking sounds. Usually the staff will play music during the scan; you can ask for your favorite selections.

PET

PET (positron emission tomography) is a way to find changes in the body's metabolism and chemical activities. It provides a color-coded picture showing how the body functions. It does this by following an injection, called a tracer, of a harmless radioactive glucose as it travels like a homing device through the body, collecting in areas where there may be a mass or tumor. If a tumor is cancerous, the PET scan causes the picture on the screen to light up where there is a "hot spot"-- a mass that is burning energy (metabolizing) at a faster rate than normal tissue.

Things to know when going for your PET scan:

- Follow clothing guidelines in CHAPTER FIVE, How to Prepare For Tests.
- You should not to eat or drink for four hours before the test, but you may take medications with water.
- It is important for you to be relaxed and very still during this procedure. Feel free to ask the nurse for a mild sedative if necessary. Remember that deep breathing is always helpful for relaxing your body.
- The scan takes from 30 minutes to two hours and is painless.

ULTRASOUND

This test uses high frequency sound waves to produce an image of tissue on a computer screen. Radiologists sometimes use this painless method to distinguish fluid cysts from solid tumors.

GETTING TEST RESULTS

Try not to anticipate the results until you actually get them. Have a clear understanding before you leave your doctor's office of when the results will be available to you. Plan to get the results from your physician several days after your test(s). If it's possible to get the results the same day, schedule the test in the morning and the doctor's visit later in the afternoon. If it's not possible to do this, arrange a time with the nurse or PA (physician's assistant) to get your results over the telephone. If you schedule a specific time to be called for a test result and that time has passed, don't hesitate to call and inquire. It's better for you to know than to worry about the potential outcome. Try to have a support person with you when you receive your results.

Sometimes, test results are not definitive, and another set of tests may be ordered. While uncertainty can be unnerving, taking action without conclusive evidence is not necessarily wise. You may wonder why you don't have scans and tests done every month in order to get accurate diagnostic information, but that could result in false alarms and inconclusive evidence. Remember that these tests play an important role in your overall treatment plan.

CHAPTER SEVEN

Treatments

There are several different courses of treatment that your doctor may offer you. Multiple, simultaneous or consecutive treatments may be suggested, but it is ultimately your decision to determine what is the best course of action for you. What follows are brief descriptions of the most common treatments available.

CHEMOTHERAPY (Chemo)

Chemotherapy is the treatment of cancer with chemical drugs that can destroy cancer cells. Normal cells grow and die in a controlled manner every minute; however, cancer develops from a single cell that has undergone mutations in its DNA, the genetic material that carries the body's heredity signals. Healthy cells can also be harmed, and it is damage to the healthy cells that results in side effects. Your oncologist can recommend chemotherapy either before or after surgery. It is given before surgery to shrink tumors for removal or following surgery to eliminate stray cells which remain. You can ask your doctors for more detailed information on the plan chosen for your chemotherapy. Make sure to ask questions such as:

- How many treatments will I have?
- How long can I expect to be on chemotherapy?
- How long will each IV treatment take?
- Will I be admitted into the hospital or will it be done in the treatment facility?

- Will the expected side effects be temporary or can they become long term?
- Will the chemo affect other medical conditions that I may have?
- Should I have dental work completed before treatment?
- When will I know if the treatment is working?
- Will it affect my fertility?
- Can it affect the people around me?
- Can my children be harmed through sweat or saliva?
- Should I avoid breastfeeding?

Chemo can also be used to decrease the risk of cancer returning after surgery. Some drugs work better together than alone and are often prescribed in combinations. Most drugs are given intravenously (IV), but oral (by mouth) drugs may be added. Chemotherapy is used to:

- Shrink a tumor before surgery or radiation therapy (called neo-adjuvant therapy)
- Help destroy any cancer that may remain after surgery or radiation (called adjuvant therapy)
- Make radiation therapy more effective
- Assist in biological therapy
- Help destroy cancer if it recurs or metastasizes.

There are other types of cancer treatment that your doctor may choose to use such as:

- Monoclonal antibodies (Herceptin®, Cetuximab®, Rituxan®, etc.) that act to destroy cancer cells with limited side effects, (See Targeted Therapies this section).

- Interferon or Interleukin®, which can give you flu-like symptoms.

You may hear your doctor refer to a cycle or course of chemotherapy. A cycle may consist of three weekly treatments or one treatment given every 21 days. The total of several cycles is a course. Cycles of chemo allow for cancer cells to be killed in their active stage (while dividing) but may not affect resting cells. The next cycle can hit those cells that were inactive that are now actively dividing and susceptible to chemo and will die. There are some chemos that kill cells in the resting phase.

The drugs you receive will depend on:

- What type of cancer you have
- Where the cancer is located in your body
- Your age and general state of health
- The aggressiveness of your disease
- The stage of cancer (Stage I, II, III, or IV) you have. Each type of cancer is staged according to specific characteristics. In general, though, "in situ" (pre-cancerous cells) have been diagnosed at the earliest possible stage.
  - o Stage I or "local" cancers have been diagnosed early and have not spread.
  - o Stage II has spread into surrounding tissues and may have limited lymph node involvement, but not beyond the location of origin.
  - o Stage III or "regional" has spread to more nearby lymph nodes.

95

o   Stage IV or "distant" cancers have spread to other parts of the body and are the most difficult to treat.

Your chemo cocktail is specific for your body's height and weight and is custom mixed for you alone. You should not compare your dosages with other patients, especially if they are on the same protocol. Several pre-medication (like anti-nausea) drugs are given either orally or IV to help reduce the risk of adverse reactions from your chemo. The majority of reactions will happen within the first 30 minutes. You should inform your nurse immediately if you are experiencing unusual or painful occurrences.   Pre-meds have a tendency to make you very drowsy, and it's fine to sleep through the treatment. Before beginning treatment, it is important to drink plenty of fluids since hydration is good for keeping your veins open. Chemo treatments vary in side effects according to the drugs you are given; therefore, it is difficult to state what will happen to an individual. Some people respond quite well with few or no side effects; others may have a more challenging course. If, at any time, you experience extreme reactions or other unmentioned side effects, it is important that you contact your doctor. Something that seems insignificant to you could be the beginning of a serious side effect. Your physician or treatment nurse should be able to give you guidelines on what to expect. For instance, hair loss can accurately be predicted.   It is recommended that you drink plenty of fluids after treatment.

You might experience one or more of the following sensations when receiving your treatment:

- A slight burning at the injection site - let your nurse know immediately so the site can be assessed for potential leaking outside the vein (ask for a warm pack to alleviate this sensation)

- Either coldness or warmth throughout your body, lasting several minutes or the entire treatment (ask for a blanket or something cold to drink)

- An overall tingling sensation

- A chemical, metallic, salty or other strange taste in the mouth from the drugs (ask for a peppermint, other hard candy, or try using a lemon peel).

There are numerous medications available to offset many of the side effects resulting from chemotherapy. Share with your doctor and/or nurse what you are experiencing; there is no reason for you to be uncomfortable throughout this experience.

Some treatments (such as Avastin®) require a 30-40 day clearance period before surgery. This drug impairs the body's ability to heal. Patients who are taking Avastin® would have to be off of it at least two months before proceeding with surgery.

Clinical Trials

A clinical trial is a research study conducted to evaluate a new treatment for cancer patients. It is designed to address specific research questions. Each clinical trial only enrolls patients who meet specific criteria or guidelines. Not all patients qualify to participate in clinical trials. A clinical trial may be considered when the standard course of treatment has not been effective. Even though you may qualify to participate in a clinical trial, the choice to do so is completely up to you. Prior to deciding, you should understand:

- What is the purpose of the study?
- What exactly does the study involve?
- What tests and treatments will be administered?
- What are the side effects and risks?
- What are the costs, if any?
- Will your insurance cover the treatment and/or drugs?

The sponsor of the trial will usually pay for the drug(s) and special tests required. It's normally up to the patient to pay for routine care, outpatient visits, hospital stay (if required), travel and any other expenses. You need to have a clear understanding from the healthcare team about what costs are covered by your insurance before joining a trial. You can contact the Cancer Information Service (CIS) at 1-800-4-CANCER (1-800-422-6237) to request information about what clinical trials are being offered around the country for different types and stages of cancer. See the Resource section for additional information.

Trial phases

Most clinical research that involves the testing of a new drug progresses in an orderly series of steps, called phases. This allows researchers to ask and answer questions in a way that results in reliable information about the drug and protects the patients. It is important for you to understand that since the treatments are experimental, outcome and side effects are not always foreseeable.

Clinical trials are usually classified into one of three phases:

Phase I – These first studies in people evaluate how a new drug should be given (by mouth, injected into the blood, or injected into the muscle), how often, and what dose is safe. It can involve patients with different tumor types to see how the treatment works on various tumors.

Phase II – This phase trial continues to test the safety of the drug, and begins to evaluate how well the new drug works. A Phase II study will focus on a particular type of cancer.

Phase III – These studies test a new drug, a new combination of drugs, or a new surgical procedure in comparison to the current standard. A participant will usually be assigned to the standard group or the new group at random (called randomization), which means patients may not receive the experimental drug and may not know which treatment they are given during a blinded trial. In double-blinded studies, neither the doctor nor the patient know which treatments are being given until the end of the trial. Phase III trials often enroll 300-5,000 patients and may be conducted at many doctors' offices, clinics, and cancer centers nationwide.

Phase IV – This phase follows FDA approval. It involves further investigation of how best to use the drug. This phase expands to thousands of patients from a wide range of facilities.

TARGETED THERAPIES

Targeted therapy for cancer is using treatment options that attack cancer cells without damaging normal cells. Since cancer cells divide rapidly, cancer treatment has focused in the past primarily on killing rapidly dividing cells. Some normal cells divide quickly too, however, and are damaged along with the cancer cells, thus causing multiple side effects. Each type of targeted therapy works differently, but they all interfere with the ability of the cancer cell to divide, to grow, to repair, and/or to communicate with other cells. Targeted therapies can be divided into three general categories: 1) those which focus on internal components and functions of the cell, 2) ones that target the receptors on the outside parts of the cell; and 3) drugs that target blood vessels that supply oxygen to the cell. Targeted therapies are not a total replacement for traditional treatment options, but are proving to be effective in combination with other therapies. For specific information on Targeted Therapies, please visit our website at www.findingthecanincancer.com.

Monoclonal Antibodies

Antibodies are part of the immune system that defends against disease. An antibody is a protein produced by white blood cells in response to bacteria or viruses entering the body. Usually the body makes it own antibodies when an infection occurs. Monoclonal antibodies have been developed for the treatment of cancer when our bodies need help with boosting our naturally made antibodies. They are designed to recognize specific proteins on cancer cells.

EGFR Inhibitors

Anti-EGFR treatments are one of the most widely studied approaches to cancer treatment. While these agents avoid many of the side effects associated with chemotherapy, they are not without side effects of their own. EGFR is found on many tumor types as well as on normal skin cells. Blocking EGFR can lead to adverse skin reactions, including rash, skin dryness and nail changes. Some studies of anti-EGFR have shown that patients who develop a rash may have a better response and longer survival times than patients who do not.

Enzyme Inhibitors

Enzyme inhibitors block enzymes inside the cancer cells. Some of the newer drugs are designed block multiple enzymes.

Proteasome Inhibitors

Proteasome inhibitors block a group of enzymes known as proteasomes which help to regulate cell function including cell death. They can stop the growth of cancer cells and allow the cells to die in a process called programmed cell death.

Antiangiogenesis

Antiangiogenesis is the process of stopping the formation of new blood vessels. Cancer cells, like all cells, need blood vessels in order to grow and spread. Most antiangiogenesis drugs work by preventing the first step in the formation of new blood vessels, which may help prevent new tumors from growing and may also help to shrink large tumors by cutting off their blood supply.

One of the most important proteins in new blood vessel growth, for example, is vascular endothelial growth factor (VEGF). Although this protein is not made in large amounts by normal cells, it is secreted by some cancer cells into surrounding areas, thus promoting new blood vessel formation. Some new anti cancer drugs are used to attack the VEGF pathway. Most

101

antiangiogenesis drugs have only mild side effects and the long-term side effects are still unknown. These drugs are often used in combination with other treatments.

PICC Lines

(Peripherally Inserted Central Catheter)

A PICC is a temporary alternative to a surgically implanted device such as a portacath or Hickman catheter. It eliminates the need for multiple needle sticks each time you have a treatment. The PICC is inserted like an IV into a vein near the bend of the elbow. After the needle is in place, a small soft catheter (small flexible tube) with a guide wire is passed through the needle into a large blood vessel. The needle and guide wire are removed and only the flexible catheter remains in place. An x-ray of your chest will be done immediately to check that the catheter has been correctly positioned. The PICC can remain in place for several to many weeks and should not limit your normal activities. Your nurse will explain how to protect the PICC while showering. Because the PICC is exposed outside of the skin, it should NOT be submerged in water. It is secured with a transparent dressing, which is changed weekly by a nurse. The first dressing change will take place 24 hours after the PICC is placed for examination of the site. A secure sterile dressing will reduce the chance of catheter complications or infection. *(Helpful Hint: Try using Glad Press n' Seal® over the area to keep it clean and dry between dressing changes.)* When not in use, the PICC will require a flush with heparin solution to keep it open. Your nurse will teach you or a family member how to do this.

✔ A tunneled catheter (such as Hickman®) is most commonly used for bone marrow transplant treatment and total parenteral nutrition. This treatment requires external care, like dressing changes and flushing.

Port (Portacath)

There's no getting around being stuck with needles and getting one stick is always preferable to many. After several treatments, veins can become weak, and a port is the ideal solution. There are several different types of ports, but the most common is a single access port. Ports are also placed in the abdomen (peritoneal) or head (intrathecal) for specific kinds of cancer (ovarian and central nervous system, respectively).

A single access port is an implantable device that makes it much easier to draw blood for tests and much safer to administer chemotherapy. It consists of a catheter (small flexible tube) that is placed in a large vein and connected to a "port" about the size of a quarter. The port is placed under the skin of your upper chest. Once inserted, it is recommended that the port not be removed until the likelihood of a cancer recurrence is minimal.

The implantation process is an outpatient procedure, often done the day of your next scheduled treatment. The port is accessed with a needle during the implantation process, and your treatment follows this procedure. Sometimes you may get the port placed before treatment day. The surgical procedure takes about one hour under general anesthesia, is relatively painless (maybe uncomfortable) and the area will be tender for approximately three weeks. A port does not require daily home care, but does require a flush every four to six weeks.

When you go in for your treatment, the nurse will access your port and be able to get vital blood information that will determine if your counts are at an acceptable level. The port will remain accessed and if your blood counts are good, you will then be able to receive your chemo with only one stick. In particular drug protocols, a port cannot be used; check with your doctor.

Unlike when searching for a vein, the port area can be numbed with a freezing spray to reduce discomfort. For some patients it isn't necessary to freeze the area because the stick is minimal. Having a port doesn't change your normal activities. You can bathe, swim and even scuba dive if you'd like. It can be removed as soon as the treatment protocol is completed, but some ports have been used for up to ten years.

Ports are especially beneficial in people who have had lymph nodes removed in their armpit (axilla) area and only one arm is available for labs, IV's, blood pressure, etc.

A word of caution: a small percentage of people have developed infections, blood clots, and other complications after placement of ports, but the majority of users have been very satisfied.

RADIATION

Radiation therapy, frequently used in the treatment of cancer, involves the use of penetrating beams of high-energy waves that easily kill the rapidly growing cancer cells. A specifically calibrated amount of radiation is directed at the tumors or areas of the body where cancer is present. Getting radiation is very much like getting an x-ray, and you can be assured that you will not "glow," become radioactive, or give off radiation from treatment. Normal cells are, however, affected by radiation and although many of them recover from its effects, the cancer cells do not. Since the radiation passes through the skin, it will be affected. You will most likely be given skin care guidelines or information by your radiation nurse; if not, be sure to ask. Fatigue and skin sensitivity or irritations are the most common radiation therapy side effects (see Skin Care and Fatigue in PART IV). Other side effects will depend on the area being treated. For example, if the area being treated is the mouth, stomach or intestine your appetite may be affected. These are some things to remember during your radiation treatments:

- Wear soft comfortable clothing if the treated area will be in contact with clothing.
- Check with your doctor or nurse regarding the use of any lotions or skin care products.
- Do not put anything hot or cold on the treated area, such as heating pads or ice packs.
- Avoid rubbing or scratching the treated area.
- Stay out of the sun.
- Wash with lukewarm water and a mild soap or cleansing lotion. Do not wash off the locator markings.
- Do not put any lotion on your skin prior to treatment or within an hour or two afterwards.

External radiation therapy is usually administered for five consecutive days a week for six to seven weeks. If you do not live within a reasonable commuting distance from the facility where you will be treated, you may need to make arrangements for a local place to stay. Ask to speak to the oncology social worker or radiation nursing staff for housing information. Even if you live locally, you may not able to drive yourself, and arranging for daily transportation can sometimes be difficult. In some areas the American Cancer Society has a service called the Road to Recovery, through which volunteers provide transportation for patients to appointments and treatment clinics.

Prior to starting your treatment you will undergo a process called *simulation.* You will be required to lie very still on an examining table in a room with a large x-ray machine, which will be used to define the field on your body to be radiated. CT scans or other imaging tests may also be done to provide needed information. It is essential that you be in the exact same position each time you receive a treatment. To insure accuracy, a body mold may be made for the area to be radiated. Your skin will be marked at the treatment site with a tattoo or permanent colored ink dots. Take care when bathing not to wash off these markings. If they begin to fade, tell your radiation therapist. The simulation can take from a half-hour to two hours. Treatment will begin a few days later.

Depending on the area being treated, you may need to change into a hospital gown. You will be in the treatment room about 15 to 20 minutes, but you are only receiving radiation for one to five minutes. There is no sensation while receiving radiation. You will be alone in the room while receiving the radiation, but you are being viewed on a TV monitor. The machines are large and look intimidating, but rest assured that you are in the hands of trained professionals. Be sure to discuss any concerns you have with the radiation therapist or the nurse. Typically, you will receive your treatment at the same time each day, and you will see your physician once a week.

Intraoperative radiation involves radiation during surgery. A surgeon first removes as much of the tumor as possible; then a large dose of radiation is directed at the area from which the tumor was removed and the surrounding area. This is sometimes followed by external radiation therapy.

Internal radiation therapy or Brachytherapy places radioactive material in a catheter or tube directly into the affected area. This provides a higher total dose of radiation in a shorter time. Brachy treatments require hospitalization and close monitoring.

SRS (Stereotactic Radiosurgery)

SRS is a treatment that uses high-energy x-rays to treat cancerous as well as non-cancerous diseases in the brain.

Prior to the day of SRS you will have an MRI scan. This is done to provide the team with precise imaging of the brain.

The treatment involves delivery of a single high dose of radiation that converge on the tumor. A brace-like device is used to keep the head completely still so the radiation is targeted and minimizes radiation to healthy brain tissue. There are some things to know about the procedure:

- You will be asked to maintain your regular diet. This will help you to avoid nausea or fainting.

- Be sure to ask your physician about whether to take any normal medications on the day of treatment, and bring those medicines with you to treatment.

- Tell your physician if any of the following apply to you: 1) you take medicine by mouth or insulin to control diabetes; 2) you are allergic to IV contrast material, shellfish or iodine; 3) you have a pacemaker, artificial heart valve, defibrillator, brain aneurysm clips, implanted pumps or chemotherapy ports, neurostimlulators, eye or ear implants, stents, coils or filters 4) you suffer from claustrophobia.

- SRS is usually an outpatient procedure, but be prepared to wait! It is an all day treatment. Wear comfortable clothing, bring snacks and something to read or do while you wait. You will need to have a family member or friend accompany you and drive you home.

After an IV has been started, a head frame or "halo" needs to be placed on the skull. There are four simultaneous injections of anesthesia to the head to be able to place the halo for accuracy. After placement of the halo, a CT scan is taken to merge with the MRI for exact locations of the lesion(s). The treatment lasts 15-45 minutes depending on the sites to be treated. The head frame will be removed and you will be given discharge orders and allowed to go home. Hair loss may occur at the treatment site.

You will have another MRI in approximately three months to follow the progress of this procedure.

SURGERY

Surgery is the oldest form of cancer treatment and can be very effective in treating some kinds of cancer. Although it isn't an option for everyone, you are likely to undergo some type of surgery as a cancer patient.

Besides being used for primary tumor removal, surgery can be performed for:

- Diagnosis (biopsy) or staging
- Implanting a device (port) to deliver drugs, or implanting radioactive seeds to deliver radiation to internal tumors
- Removal of other tumors
  - o Residual – tumors which are left smaller after chemotherapy
  - o Metastatic – spread to other organs
  - o Recurrent – tumors that recur at the original sites
- Symptom relief (stopping pain or bleeding, bowel obstruction, etc.)
- Reconstruction.

If you are going to have any type of surgery, you need to know some things to help you prepare. Every surgery is different, and the preparation will vary according to what is being done and the anesthesia you will have. These are some questions to ask before surgery:

- Will my surgery be outpatient (done in office or clinic) or inpatient (in hospital)?

- What will be done during the operation?
- Is there an illustration or photograph that will help me understand?
- What type of anesthesia will I receive?
  - o Local (which is used for numbing specific limited regions of the body)
  - o Regional/Block (used to numb a region of the body like an arm or leg)
  - o General (patient is asleep).
- Will I need to consider banking my own blood for surgery (autologous blood transfusion), or should I have family members donate in the event I need a transfusion?
- Will I need to go to intensive care?
- Will I likely have drains or catheters after the procedure?
- What (if any) is the anticipated hospitalization time?
- When will I be able to resume normal activities?
- Will I need rehabilitative therapy such as physical therapy or occupational therapy?
- When do I need to schedule a follow-up appointment?

Here are some suggestions to help prepare you for surgery:

- Stop smoking before your operation; this will help to prevent respiratory complications during anesthesia and in the postoperative period. Any length of time not smoking helps!
- If you take medication (prescription, herbal, or over-the-counter), find out from your doctor if you should keep taking it before or after the procedure (for example, aspirin can cause excessive bleeding).

- Follow special diet restrictions or take iron supplements if your doctor recommends them.

- Try not to overexert yourself, and get plenty rest in the days before your operation.

- Make sure that you arrange for a family member or friend to take you home after surgery and help with your immediate recovery.

- Reduce stress as much as possible.

Pre-Surgical Visit

The pre-surgical visit is usually one or two days before surgery. You will have an EKG (painless heart tracing), blood and urine tests. A nurse will weigh you and take your blood pressure. You should be prepared to answer lots of questions, some of which will include the following:

- What are the prescription medications you are taking and the dosages?

- What non-prescriptions drugs, vitamins, or herbal supplements are you taking and the dosages?

- Do you have allergies to any food or drugs?

- Have you had anesthesia before, and if so, were you allergic to any anesthetic drug?

- Have you had any previous blood transfusions?

- Do you have a medical history of diabetes, stroke, heart, lung, kidney, or liver disease?

- Do you drink alcohol on a daily basis?

You will also be required to arrange insurance information, and you will be required to sign an *informed consent form* which indicates you give your permission for the surgery.

The Day Before Surgery

- Do not smoke! Nicotine causes constriction of small arteries and causes respiratory complications.
- Do not eat or drink anything after midnight. The stomach needs to be empty so that food won't be vomited or inhaled into the lungs during the operation.
- When emptying your bowels before surgery, use petroleum jelly around your anus to prevent rawness.
- Don't chew gum after midnight.
- Complete any special preparations your surgeon has prescribed.
- Take only medicines your surgeon has told you to take.
- Bathe, shower, and shave the night before surgery.

The Day of Surgery

- Do not swallow any water when brushing your teeth.
- Do not wear any makeup, lipstick, or nail polish.
- Do not wear contacts.
- Wear loose fitting, comfortable clothes and shoes.
- If you have long hair, tie it back loosely or braid it.
- Leave all valuables at home (jewelry, money).

Things To Bring the Day of Surgery

- Bring a container for any glasses, dentures or hearing aids, and make sure they are labeled with your name and/or given to a family member.

- If you have asthma, bring your inhaler.

- You might want to pack a small bag and include: ✔ a robe, which opens all the way up the front ✔ slide-in slippers ✔ your toiletries ✔ A small comfortable pillow and light blanket ✔ some lip balm for dry lips after surgery ✔ a moisturizer ✔ a pen and small pad of paper ✔ a good book or magazines.

- Remember to bring any forms or reports your doctor has asked you to bring.

- Bring with you a copy of your advanced directives (see, Chapter 12) and insurance card.

What to Expect Upon Arrival

- You will sign in at the registration desk.

- Visitors are usually limited to two, and they must also register.

- If you are already a patient in the hospital, you will be wheeled down to surgery.

- If you are an outpatient, you will be called to the operating area and you will be given a hospital gown, cap and booties to wear. You will place your clothes in a bag to be given to your family members or sent to your room after surgery.

- You will be taken to a "holding room" and put into a hospital bed before going to the operating room.

- Your anesthesiologist may come to see you to explain procedures or answer questions.

- An IV (intravenous drip) will be started and you will be connected to various monitoring devices.

- You will be taken to the operating room.

Immediately After Surgery

- You will go to the recovery room following surgery. It's also known as the PACU (post-anesthesia care unit). Specially trained nurses will monitor you carefully and will administer pain medication.

- While you are in the PACU, the surgeon will meet with your family or friends to give them a surgery update and answer their questions about your condition.

- When the PACU nurse is satisfied that your condition is stable, you will be discharged and go home or to your hospital room.

- Most patients spend at least two hours in the recovery room; it might be longer depending on the type of operation.

Recovery from Surgery

- If you've received only a local anesthetic, you may be allowed to go home shortly after the procedure.

- You must not drive, operate machinery or make any major decisions for the first 24 hours after surgery.

- If you had general anesthesia, after you leave the recovery room and are taken to your hospital room, you will not feel fully awake for several hours while the effects of the anesthesia gradually wear off.

- You might have a tube coming out of the incision site (a drain), which allows excess fluid that collects at the surgical site to leave the body.

- It is likely that you will have a tube running from your bladder (a catheter) into a bag by the side of the bed. This drains your urine until you are able to urinate on your own.

- Your throat may be sore from the tube used for the anesthesia.

- Some level of pain should be expected after surgery. You will be asked about your pain on a scale from 1 (one) to 10, where 1 is mild and 10 is extreme. Try to be accurate in telling your medical team so they can provide accurate dosing of drugs to help control your pain. You might have a pain-controlled analgesic (PCA) pump which allows you to give yourself pain medication when you need it.

- You won't be allowed to have any food or water at first. Your nurse may allow you to have some ice chips, and you can request a sponge swab to clean or refresh your mouth.

- Your stomach and intestines may take several days to recover from anesthesia, and therefore you will be unable to eat until your health care team is sure that your digestive system is working. Your nurse and doctor will listen with a stethoscope for bowel sounds which indicate that things are moving again. Once this happens, you can consume liquids and then solid foods.

- You will be encouraged to get out of bed and walk as soon as possible following surgery, sometimes even the same day! This is to prevent blood clots from forming in your legs and to help regain normal bowel and bladder function. You may also wake up to find that you have compression pumps attached to your legs; this is to prevent blood clots.

- Another important part of recovery is deep breathing, which you can do to help inflate your lungs and to prevent pneumonia. You will be encouraged to cough and will most likely be given a small plastic toy-looking device called a spirometer, which helps measure how deep a breath you are taking. Even if it is painful, you need to try to cough and to breathe deeply to help clear the mucus from your lungs and prevent air sacks in your lungs from collapsing.

- Anesthesia, pain medication and decreased activity may make it difficult to achieve simple body functions. In most hospitals, for you to be released, you must have a bowel movement and urinate after the removal of your catheter.

Discharge from Hospital

Your doctor will send you home with a sheet of instructions for post-operative care; the discharge nurse will review the instructions with you.

- You will also be given various medications and prescriptions to relieve pain.

- Notify your physician immediately if any one of the following symptoms occurs, which might indicate infection of the wound:
  o Pain, swelling, redness or warmth around the incision site
  o Bleeding or drainage from the wound
  o A fever of more than 101 degrees

o   Nausea, vomiting, headache, or chills.

Before You Leave

Make sure that you understand the following:

- How to care for your wound/incision
- What your limits on activities are
- What medications to take and when, including pain medicines
- Whom to call with questions
- Whether you should do any rehabilitative exercises
- When your follow-up appointment is with your surgeon.

Ending a Treatment Phase

Ending a treatment phase can be a time of great joy and relief. At any time during the course of treatment you will know how many days of radiation or how many chemo treatments remain. When the big day finally arrives and your treatment is completed, you may be very surprised to find that accompanying the expected joy and relief is an unexpected anxiety about what will follow. You may find yourself feeling as if you are no longer dealing with the disease in an active way. You may also worry about whether enough has been done, or what will happen if the cancer returns. These worries and fears are to be expected, and they will recede as time passes. Try to keep them in perspective and to separate your overall anxiety from how you are doing physically. When the drugs have all been eliminated from your system, your life will get back to the normal you used to know. You will be scheduled to take tests for quite some time after you have finished your treatments. Discuss the follow-up with your doctor so you know what to expect. Many cancer survivors live with the uncertainty of their health after living through chemotherapy and a diagnosis of cancer. It may be a time when you realize how valuable human life really is and the measures you are willing to endure to prolong your existence.

The people you have met during this experience have touched your life in a way that you will never forget. The doctors, nurses, and staff will have become a mainstay in your experience of survival; however, they will be glad to see you go home healthy, and they are excited that you have been given a second chance to live an enjoyable life. The adjustment from seeing this team regularly during your treatment to seeing them less frequently may not be easy. Be assured that they will continue to be part of your life, and they will carefully monitor your progress. Listen to your body, so you will be aware of anything new and have it checked early. Remember that your body is not the same as before your diagnosis; it has changed, but hopefully, this means you are now cancer free.

Family and friends who have showered you with attention, casseroles, rides, etc. may now feel that everything is back to normal and leave you on your own a lot more. Getting your life back to normal is certainly an understandable goal, but life will be different now and you may need to reevaluate just what normal will be. This could be the first time you have actually had a chance to process the fact that you were diagnosed with cancer. Take time to reflect on what you have been through, evaluate where you are now, and make current plans and plans for the future. If you have not attended a support group previously, you may want to consider it now after completing your treatment. Interacting with others who are getting on with life after diagnosis and treatment can be most helpful. If you find that you are having problems with anxiety or moving on with your life, you can contact a professional counselor to help you find ways to cope and understand how you can help yourself.

Don't forget that you still have powerful resources within you - your attitude and your own immune system. Focus on things that boost your immune system: diet, exercise, meditation, visualization and other things that will improve your mind, body and spirit. Put laughter in your life and have fun. Spend time with friends and family, and do those things you always planned to do but just couldn't find the time. Make each day special – you deserve it!

PART III – Understanding Procedures

PART IV

Side Effects...

Things That Might Help

Allergies (Drug, food or sun exposure) - An allergic reaction is an overactive immune response to a foreign substance (that doesn't cause that same reaction in most people). Allergic reactions can occur after taking almost any drug and usually occur within minutes of receiving the drug. It may appear in the form of hives, itching, wheezing, coughing, runny nose, or shortness of breath within minutes or several hours after contact with the allergy-causing drug or substance. There are more severe reactions (called anaphylaxis) that can be life threatening. Inform your doctor or nurse immediately if:

- You have a known allergy to food or drugs
- You notice anything unusual during chemotherapy or after you have gotten home
- You develop a rash while taking any drug
- You have itching symptoms on the hands/palms, feet or elsewhere (many chemos can have a cumulative effect, especially with the drug carboplatin)
- You have an allergic reaction when exposed to any amount of sunlight during treatments. Remember always to use sunscreen with a SPF of 30+.

121

Anemia (See also Blood counts) - Anemia is an inadequate supply of red blood cells, which carry oxygen. Anemia causes symptoms such as fatigue, shortness of breath, rapid heartbeat, dizziness, inability to concentrate, chest pain, feeling cold, and pale skin. Most cancer patients treated with chemotherapy will experience anemia. Anemia can also make other medical problems like heart conditions worse, and it can prevent you from getting chemo treatments on schedule. It can be treated with blood transfusions or with drugs like Epogen® or Procrit® and supplemental iron tablets.

Breath, shortness of - Shortness of breath (dyspnea) is difficulty in breathing. It can make you feel as if you can't get enough air into your lungs and can be very frightening. Feeling breathless can make you feel panicky, and that anxiousness can then make you feel even more breathless. A vicious cycle is begun when you panic because the more anxious you become, the more oxygen you consume. It's important to break the cycle as soon as possible. Shortness of breath can have many causes including airway obstruction, narrowing of airways, pneumonia, fluid around the heart or lungs (see Fluid on Chest, this section), stress, or a tumor.

Some things to help when you have shortness of breath:

- Try to relax. In order to relax your shoulders and arms, try shrugging your shoulders or rotate them several times.

- Use controlled breathing. You can try pursing your lips (pucker up) and take in a normal breath through your nose.

Then exhale through your pursed lips for twice the number of seconds it took you to inhale.

- Use visualization to calm yourself (see Visualization, CHAPTER NINE).

- Use a fan to cool yourself because cooler air may be easier to breathe.

- Lower the room temperature.

- Change your position. If you are sitting, lean forward and place your elbows on your knees. If you are in bed, raise your head on pillows so you are close to sitting.

- Ask your doctor to prescribe anti-anxiety drugs or other medications to help relieve your symptoms.

Chemo-Brain - Although it is usually a temporary side effect, some patients who are receiving chemotherapy find that they have trouble concentrating, have difficulty in finding the right word, and have impaired memory. Some people refer to this as "chemo brain," and recently this condition has been validated by reported research. The problem hasn't been well studied in the past because it is harder to measure memory functions than to assess physical symptoms like nausea and vomiting. Among the many factors which can contribute to the unfocused, fuzzy-headed feeling you may experience during treatment are the following: anemia, fatigue, anxiety, depression, the effects of anesthesia and the side effects from medications. For most patients, these symptoms will resolve once treatment has been completed, and you will return to your pre-treatment brain functioning. Stress management techniques are essential to your daily routine since stress has been associated with difficulties in memory functions. Scientists believe that daily mental and physical activities help to increase the connections between brain cells and keep them active. If brain cells aren't used regularly, they and their connections will weaken. You should create your own methods of stress reduction and brain protection, since what works for one person may not work for another.

Tips for dealing with chemo-brain:

- Pay attention to what soothes and calms you, and try to remember to use these methods throughout the day.

- Find a new hobby (or retry one you used to like), such as ✔ reading ✔ working puzzles ✔ playing a musical instrument ✔ painting ✔ cooking ✔ brainteasers ✔ woodworking ✔ knitting, crocheting, or doing other needlework ✔ writing journals, poems or stories ✔ playing computer games.

- Do regular physical activity such as walking, going up and down stairs, and gardening.

- Try to remember to drink fluids; your brain needs hydration as well.

Constipation is the condition in which a person's bowels move far less frequently than normal. People who are constipated may have small, hard, dark stools, pain or discomfort or may need to strain to pass stools. Constipation is caused when too much water is absorbed from the large intestine back into the bloodstream, leaving the feces dry, hard and difficult to expel. Normal elimination varies for each person, but ideally, you should have a bowel movement each day. It is extremely common for patients undergoing chemotherapy to experience constipation, which if it not treated immediately, can lead to serious conditions such as fecal impaction and even bowel obstruction. Constipation can be one of the most uncomfortable side effects of chemotherapy and can ultimately result in the need for surgery if left untreated. Diet is one of the main factors that affect the movement of your bowels; eating high fiber and bulky food every day aids your digestion. Bran flakes, fresh or dried fruits, whole grain cereal, nuts and popcorn are good choices. Remember that you may have to drink more fluids when you increase fiber, or you may become constipated from the fiber. Other causes of constipation:

- Postponing visits to the toilet
- Using laxatives excessively (can cause your bowels to become dependent on those aids, while the natural function of your sphincter muscles decreases)
- Medications such as narcotics for pain, antidepressants, antihistamines, tranquilizers, diuretics and other drugs
- Scarring from radiation or surgery
- Emotional stress.

Things that might relieve constipation:

- Drink plenty of fluids (8 to 10 eight ounce glasses of filtered water a day).
- Exercise daily since exercise helps to regulate your body and helps your normal bodily processes to run smoothly. If you are unable to walk, there are abdominal exercises, which you

can do in bed to help your bowels to keep moving (ask your doctor).

- Take a warm bath, which can relax the sphincter muscle, as well as relieve anxiety, or use a heating pad or hot water bottle.

- Try to have a bowel movement at the same time each day.

- Don't use suppositories or enemas unless ordered by your doctor. In some cancer patients, these treatments can cause bleeding, infection or other harmful side effects. Your doctor may tell you to take a laxative, stool softener, suppository or enema. It is best to check with him/her before using any of these over-the-counter remedies. There are several brands, and your pharmacist can help you choose. Stool softeners can help keep the stool soft to avoid hemorrhoids.

Terri – A natural and gentle pain-free aid that I have had success with is called Aloelax®.

- Keep a record of all bowel movements so you can be aware of regularity problems.

- Keep your rectal area clean and dry. Use personal wipes products such as Tucks®, Cottonelle®, etc.

- Avoid cheese, chocolate, white bread and caffeinated products.

- Drink warm coffee and tea (both in moderation), hot lemon water and prune or apple juice, either warm or cold.

- You can also try *Nancy's* homemade recipe. Add 2 Tbsp of flaxseed (ground, cold-pressed) to your diet every day. You can mix it in water or juice. One of our favorite mixtures is

1/3 cup cottage cheese, 2 Tbsp ground flaxseeds, 2 Tbsp flaxseed oil, blueberries (good antioxidants) or other fruits.

- If you experience constipation, when you have a bowel movement, your anus may split and bleed. Try to use a mild lubricant like Vaseline® or Neosporin® to help soften the skin during bowel movements.

- If you have a colostomy bag, try adding baby oil to the bag. Not only is it gentle on the stoma and skin, it also helps the feces to slide out and leaves the bag clean and odor free.

- Adding an aspirin to a colostomy bag helps dissipate the odor or passed gas.

Dehydration is a condition in which you lose more fluids than you take in, and it can be a very serious condition. In addition to water loss, dehydration means loss of electrolytes such as calcium, sodium and potassium. Vital organs like the heart, brain and kidneys need balanced electrolytes to function properly. Dehydration can result from vomiting, diarrhea, infection, high fever, frequent urination, bleeding, or external causes such as hot weather, airplane travel, drinking alcohol, or not drinking enough liquids. There are three levels of dehydration: mild, moderate, and severe, which are indicated by the following symptoms:

Mild dehydration:

- Dry mouth and nose
- Feeling dizzy or light-headed
- Feeling very tired or weak

- Low urine output or darker-colored urine (more concentrated).

Moderate dehydration:

- Deep, rapid breathing
- Sunken eyes
- Skin that doesn't bounce back when you pinch it lightly and let it go.

Severe dehydration:

- Weak, rapid pulse
- Cold hands and feet
- Blue lips
- Confusion.

Treatment for dehydration:

If dehydration is related to uncontrolled nausea or diarrhea, it is important to get these symptoms under control (see Nausea, Diarrhea and Vomiting this section).

- Drink plenty of clear fluids (8-10 glasses per day) such as water, broth, Jell-O® or Gatorade®.
- If you are unable to drink enough liquids, eat ice chips (remember: it takes a lot of ice chips to equal one 8-ounce glass).
- Suck on Popsicles®.
- Eat sherbet or sorbet.
- Intravenous fluids may be necessary if you become unable to drink enough liquids to replace your body fluids.

Notify your doctor if you experience any of the symptoms listed above, in case IV fluids are needed to reverse dehydration quickly.

Depression - Feeling depressed is a common response to the diagnosis of cancer or during difficult stages of treatment. There may be periods when you feel sad and overwhelmed by what you are facing. Life is a series of challenges, and a certain degree of stress is to be expected during every phase of change in our lives. Normal stresses of everyday life, however, are compounded by cancer, and may involve additional life issues such as the following:

- Fear of pain and the unknown
- Fear of death
- Changes in life plans
- Interrupted schedules
- Different social roles and lifestyles
- Changes in body image, and self-esteem (for example, having a body part removed that will affect your sexuality)
- Changes in the way people respond to you because of your disease
- Concerns about money and legal affairs.

Feeling scared, sad or depressed is nothing to be ashamed of, and you need to recognize such feelings and monitor the degree to which you experience them. It's important, however, to distinguish between normal sadness, which lessens with time, and depression, which needs to be treated. If you have five or more of the following symptoms every day for at least two weeks, or if they are interfering with your daily activities (taking care of yourself or your children, your social life or work, etc.), ask your doctor to refer you to a specialist for an evaluation of depression:

- Feeling sad or anxious for most of the day, nearly every day
- Having trouble sleeping or spending most of the day sleeping
- Losing interest in doing things or not enjoying things you usually do (including sex)
- Having no appetite or eating constantly (weight changes)
- Feelings of overwhelming fatigue
- Feeling hopeless, helpless, worthless or guilty
- Being unable to concentrate, remember or make decisions
- Being irritable and restless
- Having thoughts of death or suicide.

Whether depression originates from cancer or from a pre-existing condition, remember that it can limit the energy that you need to focus on dealing with cancer. Even mild symptoms of depression are distressing and need to be addressed. Here are things that might help with depression:

- Share your true feelings with those who care about you. See also CHAPTER ONE.
- Join a support group or consult with a patient support volunteer.
- Exercise.
- Try to help someone else.
- Listen to beautiful music.

- Pray or meditate.

- Don't lose sight of what is good in your life, and accept the love and support of those who care about you.

- Seek professional help for possible counseling and prescription medications.

Diarrhea can easily lead to dehydration and depletion of electrolytes that can quickly become a serious condition (see Dehydration in this section). Diarrhea is a condition in which your stools are more frequent than usual, loose and watery. You may have associated gas (flatulence), bloating, cramping, abdominal pain, urgency and depletion of important electrolytes. Call your doctor if your diarrhea is severe or lasts longer than 24 hours.

Common causes of diarrhea include chemotherapy, radiation, antibiotics, other drugs, lactose intolerance, intestinal infections, and emotional disturbances.

Things to help with diarrhea:

- Try resting your bowels for 10-12 hours by drinking only clear liquids (see Nutrition, Clear Liquid Diet, this section) when you have a sudden, short-term attack of diarrhea.

- Eat frequent small meals throughout the day to avoid overloading your stomach and stimulating contractions in your digestive system. High sodium foods and high potassium foods like broth, potatoes (boiled, baked or mashed), bananas, peaches and apricots are good. Other foods that are helpful are crackers, applesauce, yogurt (especially good if diarrhea is caused by antibiotics, since yogurt can replace good bacteria in your digestive system), cooked cereals such as cream of wheat, grits, toast or white bread, pastas, rice, eggs, cottage cheese, cooked vegetables, fish, cooked or canned skinless fruit, cream cheese, skinless chicken or turkey.

- Drink plenty of liquids to replace lost fluids. Attempt to drink at least 8 eight-ounce glasses of decaffeinated fluids every day such as broth, fruit juices, Popsicles® and Jell-O®, herbal (decaf) tea, and sports drinks (which replace potassium and electrolytes).

- Milk and milk products can aggravate diarrhea because of lactose, so if your diarrhea is due to lactose intolerance, you can take lactase supplements (Lactaid®, Dairy Ease®, etc.) to help with this problem.

- Avoid eating popcorn, bran, whole grain bread and cereal, nuts, seeds, coconut, raw fruit, broccoli, cabbage, corn, cauliflower, beans, peas, spicy foods, chocolate, alcoholic and caffeinated beverages.

- Try eating one coconut macaroon in the morning and one in the evening.

- For comfort, wrap a towel around a warm water bottle or use a heating pad on your stomach, being careful not to burn skin, which may be more sensitive due to chemo or radiation.

- Use warm water or gentle wiping products such as Tucks® or Cottonelle® to help protect and clean the tissue around your anus, which can easily become irritated after each movement. Use a healing ointment or salve such as A&D ointment®, Neosporin® or a triple antibiotic ointment. Your doctor may prescribe a medication to control diarrhea and will give you instructions on how to take it.

Dizziness (See also Fainting) - Dizziness, light-headedness or "vertigo" can result from any number of medications that you take. Low blood counts and fatigue can make you light-headed. It also may be caused by dehydration, which lowers your blood pressure and makes you feel woozy or faint. You could have a problem with inflammation of your inner ear, which controls balance. All of these things can affect you at any given moment, but especially when you change position, rise quickly or move your head. It is important to notify your doctor if symptoms persist, if there is a loss of vision or hearing, or if your symptoms become more severe.

To help minimize the spinning effects:

- Drink plenty fluids, avoiding caffeine and alcohol.
- Change positions slowly, allowing your body the chance to adapt to the position change.
- Try doing vestibular exercises to get rid of your dizziness; ask your doctor for more information.

Eyes - There are some chemotherapy drugs that can cause excessively watery eyes. There are eye drops that can reduce this side effect. Some chemotherapies can result in the destruction of the tear ducts. If you start to produce excess tears, consult your oncologist first. If drops don't help, consult an ophthalmologist

133

(eye specialist) who specializes in lachrymal (tear) work. In some cases, surgery on the tear ducts to insert a small tube may be necessary to keep the tear ducts from being destroyed. For patients who suffer from excessive tearing, there are some tissue products that do not stick to your eyes and therefore, are more effective at wiping the tears. Silky Touch® tissues are more the texture of a napkin and are available in bright patterns. They can be found at drug and specialty stores; some plain white ones are in grocery stores.

What you can do to help with eye problems:

- Wear sunglasses to protect your eyes, which may be more sensitive to light.

- Have a baseline checkup with an ophthalmologist before you begin your chemotherapy.

- For symptoms such as dry eyes, try over-the-counter eye drops or ask for prescription eye drops.

- Be sure to tell your oncologist of any changes that occur after you begin your chemotherapy such as burning, blurry vision, tearing, double vision, or change in color perception, as compared to the baseline exam. Many of these changes may be reversible if they are recognized early, and your doctor can reduce or discontinue the drug that is causing the side effect.

Fainting (See also Dizziness) - Fainting can be a side effect of medications or chemotherapy and should be reported immediately to your physician. If you know that a medication you are taking can cause dizziness and fainting, do not drive an automobile or operate heavy machinery. Also, get up slowly from a sitting position to give the blood a chance to travel to your brain before you begin to walk. If you begin to feel faint, sit down and lower your head.

Fatigue (See also CHAPTER THREE, How to Let Others Help You - if you need help with normal activities due to fatigue.) - Studies have shown that fatigue is the most common side effect of cancer treatment. It can range from feeling tired most of the time to being absolutely exhausted. The fatigue experienced by a cancer patient is different from that of everyday life. It is a tiredness that can begin suddenly; it can be overwhelming and is not always relieved by rest. It can affect a person's mood and ability to do normal activities and to concentrate (see Chemo Brain in this section). Let your doctor know how fatigue is affecting your regular routine. Make a list of the activities that are causing you difficulty. There are medications that can help to offset some of the fatigue. This temporary reduction in energy will return to normal when treatments are finished and your body has had a chance to re-energize itself. Among the medical causes of fatigue are the following: the cancer process itself, chemotherapy, pain, fever, night sweats, not drinking enough fluids, electrolyte imbalance, anemia, poor nutrition, and breathing (respiratory) problems. Some things that you can do to help to deal with fatigue:

• Try to get six to eight hours of sleep every night.

- Take short naps throughout the day; a half-hour to 45 minutes is refreshing. Don't over-nap during the day or you might be unable to sleep through the night.
- Plan your activities during the day in order to pace yourself.
- Avoid doing things for long periods at a time.
- Take short breaks during difficult activities.
- Don't stand when you can sit.
- Try to do the most important and fun activities first when you have the most energy.
- Climb the stairs only when absolutely necessary.
- Wear comfortable shoes and loose fitting clothing.
- Eat a well balanced diet and small frequent meals throughout the day rather than three large ones. Cook meals when you have lots of energy and freeze them to use later.
- Drink 8 eight-ounce glasses of fluid a day; consider nutritional supplements like Boost®, Ensure® or Sustacal®.
- Bathing/showering can be tiring. Plan it for a time when you can rest afterwards (like right before bed). Let a terrycloth bathrobe do the work of drying you.
- Simplify things; move things you use frequently to low, easily accessible areas.
- If you can, alter your work schedule. Discuss your treatment schedule and the effect it might have on your work with your supervisor prior to starting treatment. Consider working fewer hours. Be realistic with your employer and yourself about work goals. Try to take time off during your treatment time. During lunch or break periods, take a nap or rest if you

can. Check to see if you are eligible for time off through the Family Medical Leave Act or other time that might be available through your employer. Use the Job Accommodation Network (800-232-9675); it is a free service that can help employers make special arrangements such as flexible hours for employees who need them.

- Remember to rest when you start feeling tired rather than waiting until you are exhausted.
- Try to keep a reasonable regular exercise routine.
- Be as active as you can without pushing yourself. You can walk, do yoga, do stretching, or swim. Try to do easier, shorter versions of activities that you enjoy.
- Listen to your body if you are tired; rest.
- Use physical therapy to help with muscle weakness.
- Try getting respiratory therapy if you are having difficulty with shortness of breath, which can make you feel very tired.
- Consider getting a temporary handicapped driver's tag if you need it to avoid too much walking.
- Try activities that are less strenuous such as reading, talking to friends or listening to music.
- Delegate tasks. It not only helps you, but family and friends feel better if they can do something to help you.

Fever is an abnormally high body temperature and is always an indication that something is wrong. The average body temperature is 98.6°F (37°C); but each person is different, and normal ranges are from 97°F to 99°F. Usually, our temperatures are lower in the morning and higher in the afternoon. The body produces fever to fight disease, and it is an especially important sign for cancer patients because it may be a signal of infection. Fevers can result in chills, headaches, exhaustion, dehydration, and seizures. Always keep a thermometer handy and be sure that you know how to use it.

- If you develop a fever over 101°, call your doctor immediately. A fever of 104° or more can be dangerous to the brain and heart. Tell your family and friends that if you develop seizures, delirium or extreme confusion that they should take you to the emergency room immediately or call 911.

- Use a digital thermometer, a strip thermometer on your forehead, or an oral thermometer, which you must leave under your tongue for three minutes before you read it.

- Do not drink, eat or smoke for at least 10 minutes before you take your temperature.

- Check with your doctor about whether to take an over-the-counter fever reducer such as acetaminophen (Tylenol®), ibuprofen (Advil®), naproxen (Napsyn ®) or salicylic acid (aspirin).

- Drink more fluids than normal because fevers can cause dehydration.

- Take a cool bath to help lower your temperature or place cold compresses on your forehead.

- Keep a record of your temperature every few hours, and note any symptoms to report to your doctor.

The American College of Physicians recommends drinking four to six, 16-ounce glasses of filtered water or other non-caffeinated beverages every 12 hours. "Feed a fever" is the old saying, and it is true. Fevers cause you to burn fuel at a higher rate, so you need more calories.

Fluid on Chest (Lungs and Heart) - Cancer and some chemotherapy may cause excessive fluid in the body, especially around the heart and lungs. Excessive fluid in the space that encases the lungs is called pleural effusion. This can cause shortness of breath, difficult breathing or fatigue. You may also notice that you are coughing when you rise up from bending down, or that you become very tired. Your doctor may order chest x-rays to determine if you have excessive fluid, and if it is significant, the fluid will have to be removed.

Nancy - You will be amazed at the difference this will make in the way you feel once it has been removed.

Things you can do to help:

- Prop yourself up to sleep, or sit at a 45° angle. Doing this allows gravity to expand the lungs and enables you to cough up phlegm.
- Stay calm, relax and try to focus on controlling your breathing since shortness of breath can cause anxiety.
- Limit your exercise.
- Drink plenty of fluids to help thin the secretions from your lungs.
- Don't drink or eat dairy products because they thicken phlegm.

- Use a humidifier to prevent airway dryness and thick mucous (be sure to clean the humidifier each day).
- Don't smoke!

Gas (Flatulence, Wind, Burping) - Gas or air in the stomach or bowels causes you to pass gas or burp.

To help prevent gas:

- Chew with your mouth closed and take small bites.
- Don't talk with your mouth full, so as not to swallow air.
- Chew your food well. (Try chewing 20 times per bite.)
- Sip drinks instead of gulping.
- Avoid gas-causing foods such as beans, broccoli, cauliflower, cabbage, and carbonated drinks.
- Do not drink with a straw.

To treat gas:

- Dissolve 2 teaspoonfuls of peppermint in a cup of hot water.
- Exercise such as walking can help.
- Take an over-the-counter medication such as Mylanta®, Phazyme®, or Beano®.
- Try aromatic bitters (found in the grocery store) to help reduce gas and its odors. Take 1-4 teaspoonfuls after meals or added to beverages and meals.
- Ask your doctor for prescription medication if the gas persists.

Hair Loss (Alopecia) - Since hair is such a visible part of one's identity, losing it can be one of the most devastating side effects of cancer. Although not all cancer treatments cause hair loss, many do, so you need to discuss this possibility with your doctor prior to starting any type of treatment. Both radiation and chemotherapy can cause hair loss. You may lose all or some of your hair on your scalp, eyebrows, eyelashes, nose, beard, and mustache. Your body hair may also thin out or disappear altogether from your armpits, arms, legs and groin.

Hair loss from radiation therapy If you are having radiation to the head, you will probably lose hair in the area that is directly radiated. Radiation to other parts of the body will not cause scalp hair loss. Ask your doctor what to expect. Hair may not grow back in the areas where you receive radiation.

Hair loss from chemotherapy Hair loss is a side effect of various treatment protocols. The type of treatment and the frequency of treatments will determine whether or not you will lose your hair. In some cases your hair may become thinner and change texture. Hair loss usually begins from 7-21 days after you start taking chemotherapy, but this also varies from person to person. Some patients experience a tingling feeling on their scalp prior to losing their hair. Usually your hair doesn't come out all at one time, but gradually over several weeks. You will notice lots of hair in your brush, on your pillow and on clothes. Once these signs appear, you may find that it is better to shave your head or cut the hair very short before it falls out (this helps to prevent clogged shower and sink drains and the nuisance of having loose hair everywhere). Having a plan regarding hair loss can give you a sense of control. Some patients have planned intimate hair-shaving parties, inviting friends and family to join them in the experience. They listen to music, enjoy refreshments, laugh, and cry and make the best of the expected unpleasant event.

Some things that might help when you lose your hair:

- Use gentle hair products such as baby shampoo to prevent dryness of the scalp.

- Brush your hair with a baby brush gently to protect your tender scalp.

- Use a nightcap on cold nights or in air conditioning, or wear a hairnet, soft cap or turban at night to collect any loose hair.

- Try to avoid nylon pillowcases, which can irritate your scalp.

- Avoid perfumed deodorants if you have lost underarm hair (baby powder or cornstarch is a good substitute).

- Rub cocoa butter or massage oil on a baldhead - it feels good and keeps it moisturized.

- Keep your scalp protected with SPF 30+ sunscreen at all times if you decide not to wear a cap.

Head coverings - Some patients prefer to wear hats, scarves, turbans, bandanas or baseball caps when they lose their hair. These come in many colors, and some are soft and comfortable. You can add a small wiglet and attach it to the front to make it look more natural. Remember to choose your most flattering colors for hats and scarves. (Wearing white may make you appear too pale.) You should focus on looking your very best, as this will make you feel better about yourself while you are going through this experience. Color makes you look healthier. Wearing your best colors will brighten your look as well as your

142

outlook. You may want to focus on wearing pretty, colorful earrings to add some pizzazz. Some patients prefer to wear nothing on their heads at all, and they can look quite beautiful and striking. Do whatever makes you feel comfortable.

Finding a Wig – (See CHAPTER EIGHT Looking and Feeling Better)

When Your Hair Grows Back - Your hair will begin to grow back about a half inch per month. You can begin to see some stubble growth from six weeks up to four months after your last treatment. It may be a different texture or color from your original hair, but it will usually return to normal after some time. You should wait until it is about three inches long before you resume coloring or bleaching. If you have a tender scalp or sores, do not bleach or color your hair until the conditions have healed. Semi-permanent hair color is less damaging to the hair than permanent hair color.

Hand and Foot Syndrome   also Neuropathy, this section) -
Hand and foot syndrome is known medically as PPE (Plantar/palmar erythroidysesthesia) and with some chemo can cause symptoms including tingling, pain, soreness, loss of sensation, swelling and skin peeling on the fingers and palms of the hands and the soles of the feet. Care of the feet is always important, but especially so during chemotherapy. Things that you can do to help:

- Wear cotton socks and gloves to reduce friction and avoid heat exposure (this also helps if your nylons adhere to the peeling soles of your feet).

- Use warm or tepid, not hot, water when bathing.

- Keep hands and feet clean and dry; apply moisturizer gently.

- Stay off your feet as much as possible.

- You can use Noni® oil to help relieve burning on the soles of the feet and palms if they become tender and begin to peel. (This product can be found on the internet.)

- You can try emu oil with MSM (known as Blue Stuff®) on the bottoms of the feet as often as you can to help healing.

- Wear non-restricting, comfortable shoes.

- If burning occurs, try immersing your feet/hands in ice water or use cool packs.

- Try using bags of frozen peas or corn, etc. as ice packs because they conform to your feet.

- Talk to your doctor about using vitamin B6.

Headache (See also Pain) - Call your doctor immediately if you experience a headache that lasts more than 24 hours and if it is not relieved with normal headache medication.

Hemorrhoids are swollen, inflamed veins around the anus and lower rectum usually caused by straining to move stools. Contributing factors include aging, chronic constipation, diarrhea, and radiation therapy.

- Treat hemorrhoids by sitting in warm tub baths several times a day for about 10 minutes at a time.

- Use a hemorroidal cream or suppositories, like PreparationH®.

144

- Try not to strain excessively or use force when rubbing or cleaning around the anus because it may cause irritation, itching and bleeding.

- Keep the rectal area very clean after each bowel movement. Use Tucks® or wet wipes such as Cottenelle®.

- Try to keep your stools soft so that they can pass easily with little straining. Empty your bowels as soon as possible after the urge occurs.

- Increase fiber in your diet by eating fruits, vegetables and whole grains and take a bulk stool softener or fiber supplement (Metamucil®, Citrucel®, Ducolax® or Aloelax®).

- Drink 6 to 8 eight ounce glasses of filtered water a day.

Hot Flashes usually start on the chest, neck and face and last between three to six minutes; they can happen several times a day. Some women also experience insomnia along with the rush of heat and sweating in association with hot flashes.

The following tips can be helpful:

- Effexor®, Zoloft® and Paxil® are prescribed anti-depressants that are very effective in reducing the number and intensity of hot flashes; ask your doctor if you feel it is necessary.

- There are some herbal remedies like black cohosh that may help to relieve hot flashes; discuss with your doctor.

- Try to avoid anything hot like rooms, food, tubs, showers, saunas and weather.

- Drink cold juice or filtered water to help reduce the intensity of the flush, and to keep hydrated.

- Avoid caffeine, alcohol and spicy foods.

- Keep ice water or an ice pack by your bed for nighttime sweats and flashes.

- Use cotton sheets, lingerie and clothing - they are less likely to trap the heat.

- Dress in layers that can be removed at the first sign of a hot flash. Avoid wool or turtleneck sweaters.

- Try wearing slip-on shoes so you can quickly put your feet on cool floor.

Indigestion (See also Nausea) - There are many prescription and over-the-counter products for acid reflux, indigestion, and heartburn such as Mylanta®, Zantac®, Tagamet®, etc.

Terri – Gaviscon® is the only over-the-counter product that worked for me; when chewed, it foams in your mouth and coats your esophagus and stomach.

Difficulty swallowing (dysphagia) occurs when food/liquid stops in the esophagus. This happens most often because of consistent stomach acid reflux (backing up) into the esophagus. Over time, the reflux causes irritation and a narrowing (stricture) of the esophagus. Food and eventually liquids feel like they are sticking in the middle and lower chest. There may be chest discomfort or even sharp pain. If you have an especially sensitive stomach, get a prescription from your doctor to help relieve discomfort. (See Throat, this section.)

Infections - Chemotherapy can lower your white blood cell counts, and since white cells are your infection fighters, you are at higher risk for all kinds of infections. While colds and flu are the most common infections, they are not the only ones. Besides respiratory infections, you can get bacterial, viral, or fungal infections as well.

Symptoms of infection that you should report to your doctor without delay include:

- A temperature of 101°F or higher
- Diarrhea for more than two days
- Severe chills, shivering or night sweats
- Burning or pain while urinating
- Headache, neck stiffness
- Severe coughing or sore throat
- Redness, swelling or puss oozing around a wound, sore, boil or pimple
- Joint pain or chest pain
- Shortness of breath or difficulty breathing
- Unusual blood or discharge in urine (cloudy) or stool (excessive mucous).

Things you can do to prevent getting an infection:

- Wash your hands thoroughly with soap and water before and after meals and visits to the bathroom.
- Use liquid soap and dry with paper towels to avoid transmission of bacteria.

- Bathe or shower daily; clean carefully between skin folds and especially in the groin area. Pat your skin dry or use a hair dryer on low heat to dry your body.

- Avoid razor cuts by using electric shavers.

- Don't touch your face, and keep your fingers out of your eyes, nose and mouth.

- Clean your teeth with a soft bristle brush and gently floss between your teeth.

- Be careful with your nail cuticles; use a cream remover instead of cutting.

- Be sure to clean well under your nails and around any jewelry.

- Be gentle with your skin; protect it from burns, scrapes, punctures and cuts.

- Do not squeeze or pick pimples.

- Don't share personal items that could have germs such as towels, hairbrushes, combs, razors, toothbrushes, or drinking glasses.

- Avoid exposure to sick people and crowded areas.

- Cook your food thoroughly and wash all fruits and vegetables well.

- Don't handle kitty litter and avoid bird and other animal feces (let others clean the cages).

- Avoid gardening (if you do garden, use gloves and mask to avoid breathing spores, etc.).

- Prevent bug bites.

- Keep out of the sun and wear sunscreen (SPF 30+) if you go out. Blistered skin, which can peel, allows infection to enter.

Women

- Be especially careful to avoid feminine hygiene sprays, tampons and sanitary pads with deodorants.

- Remember to change tampons frequently during menstruation and use sanitary pads whenever possible.

- Remember, always wipe from front to back after bowel movements to prevent contamination of the vagina with stool.

- Avoid rough sexual intercourse and use proper lubrication during intercourse to prevent injuring the delicate tissues in the genital area.

- Use birth control other than IUD's.

- Wear cotton underwear and always avoid tight clothing.

- Vaginal infections can be especially troublesome for women during chemotherapy because hormonal balance is altered and resistance to infection is lowered. When taking antibiotics for a bacterial infection, be sure to eat yogurt or drink acidophilus milk or take acidophilus tablets. These can be found in the drug store and do not require a prescription. These measures will help restore the good bacteria (which are killed by the antibiotic) needed to prevent yeast infections.

Ask your doctor about whether or not you should be immunized against certain infectious diseases.

Itching (Pruritis) - Itching is the sensation that causes you to want to scratch, and can be the cause of great distress and discomfort. Scratching can cause skin irritation and breaks in the skin surface that can lead to infection. Itching is a symptom of a problem; it's not a disease. Be sure to tell your doctor if you are experiencing this symptom.

Some of the things that might cause itching are:

- Chemotherapy drugs, hormonal agents and immunotherapies
- Radiation therapy or the combination of chemo and radiation
- An allergic reaction
- Some painkillers, antibiotics, tranquilizers, anti-inflammatories, and other drugs
- Emotional distress
- Infection
- For breast patients – you may experience phantom itching on or near the area of your mastectomy. When scratched, no relief occurs. Nylon or lace can sometimes cause itching. Try changing the fabric next to the affected areas.

Some suggestions for things you can do to help:

- Interrupt the itch-scratch-itch cycle by putting a cool washcloth or ice over the itching area.
- Take warm or tepid baths that last no longer than one hour every day. More frequent bathing and hot tubs can remove natural oils in skin and cause itching. After bathing, apply fragrance-free, alcohol-free, menthol-free, preservative-free emollient moisturizer while your skin is slightly wet. These lotions can seal water into your skin. Use mild soaps such as

Dove®, Ivory®, pure castile soap, glycerin soap or Neutrogena® instead of the harsher brands. Soak in a tubful of colloidal bath treatment containing powdered oatmeal (such as Aveeno®), bran, or starch.

- Avoid bubble baths and perfumed powders, which can irritate the skin.

- Drink plenty of liquids (8 eight-ounce glasses each a day) because skin gets most of its moisture from blood vessels in the tissues below the skin.

- Cornstarch is an effective treatment for dry skin caused by radiation treatment; make sure that it is not applied to moist surfaces because it can cause fungal growth in such areas (like the vagina, anus, and skin folds).

- In cold weather, wear gloves, a scarf, and face covering to protect your skin from chafing.

- Keep your skin moist by using hydrated creams and lotions, which prevent dryness.

- Don't overheat your home since heat is thought to make itching worse. Heat can also reduce humidity, further aggravating itchy skin. Use a room humidifier (but change the water everyday and keep it clean).

- Stay indoors as much as possible during hot and dry weather.

- Use a sunscreen with SPF 30+ when you go outside (sunburn will cause your skin to itch).

- Make sure that all detergent is washed out thoroughly from your clothing; residue from detergent and fabric softeners may make itching worse. The National Cancer Institute advises adding vinegar during the rinse cycle (one teaspoon per quart of water) to help neutralize these residues.

- Use cotton clothing that is loose-fitting and lightweight.
- Cover your bed with cotton sheets and cotton flannel blankets.
- Use hypoallergenic or natural cosmetics.
- Avoid all perfumes, aftershaves and soaps, which contain alcohol and can dry out the skin, causing itching.
- Try to avoid eating spicy or very hot foods or drinking hot beverages or alcohol, which can cause blood vessels to enlarge and encourage itching.
- Sometimes medications by mouth may be necessary to relieve itching. These may include antihistamines, such as Benedryl®, Atarax®, antibiotics, sedatives, tranquilizers, and antidepressants. Ask your doctor for suggestions.

Lips can become extremely dry and chapped from certain drug therapies and from dehydration. It is very important to drink 8-10 eight ounce glasses of water every day. There are many lip preparations which help prevent or repair chapped lips, including Vaseline®, Blistex®, Chap Stick®. Emu oil lip treatments, Zum Kiss® and Burt's Bees®, which are natural, can be found in your health food store. Cold sores (fever blisters) caused by the herpes virus can be activated by stress. There are new medications now available that can greatly reduce the duration and extent of the sores (prescription acyclovir or over-the-counter Abreva®). Ask your doctor for a prescription if you are prone to fever blisters so you can use this medicine at the onset of the outbreak.

Lymphedema - (Swelling of the arms and legs) Lymphedema is an accumulation of fluid in the tissues that results in swelling in the arm(s), leg(s), or in other parts of the body. It happens when the lymphatic vessels are damaged or removed. Lymphedema can develop as a result of surgery, radiation, infection or trauma. When surgery requires the removal of lymph nodes, it can put patients at risk for developing lymphedema. This can happen immediately after surgery, or it may take weeks, months, or even years to develop. Having chemo on the arm on which surgery was performed can result in lymphedema. Changes in air pressure during airplane travel can cause lymphedema in cancer patients who have had surgery. If your flight is longer than one hour, you should get up at least once every hour or more, and walk through the aisle to prevent lymphedema. Radiation is known to damage healthy lymph nodes and vessels, causing scar tissue to form and restricting the flow of the lymphatic fluid. When receiving radiation treatments, be careful to monitor skin changes such as increased temperature, discoloration and blistering. If lymphedema goes untreated, fluid continues to accumulate, leading to an increase of swelling and a hardening of the tissue. This condition should be reported to your doctor immediately. Faster recovery occurs when lymphedema is discovered early, so you should be aware of the early signs of swelling and tell your doctor about any of the following symptoms:

- Tightness in the arm or leg

- Rings or shoes that become too tight

- Weakness in the arm or leg

- Pain, aching, or heaviness in the arm or leg

- Redness, swelling, or signs of infection.

To help prevent the onset of lymphedema, consider the following suggestions:

- Don't allow anyone to take your blood pressure with a cuff or get needle sticks on the affected arm.

- Wear a compression sleeve, especially during air travel.

- Avoid extreme temperature changes, (such as hot baths, hot tubs, saunas, heating pads, heat-producing gels, and heated massages and ice packs).

- Don't carry heavy objects and avoid pushing or pulling with the affected arm or shoulder.

- Wear loose clothing.

- Wear your watch or bracelets on the unaffected wrist.

- Avoid alcohol and tobacco products.

- Be careful cutting nails; don't get manicures that cut the skin around the nails (cuticles).

- Don't use chemical hair removers under arms or on legs; use an electric razor instead of a safety razor.

- Wear protective gloves when gardening or doing chores and always use oven mitts when handling hot food.

- Use gloves when you wash dishes or hand-wash clothes.

- Keep affected hand and arm extra clean without using harsh soaps; try using Dove® with moisturizers.

154

- Dry your skin in a gentle patting manner, paying special attention to creases in-between fingers and toes.

- Try antibiotic ointment for insect bites and use alcohol-free bug repellants when outdoors.

- Rest your arm or leg in an elevated position above your heart with support from several pillows.

- Use a thimble when you sew.

- Apply sunscreen SPF30+ to prevent sunburn.

- Take frequent breaks when scrubbing, mopping, cleaning, or while doing other vigorous or repetitive activities, especially if your arm feels tired, heavy or achy.

- Don't cross your legs when sitting or sit in one position for more than 30 minutes.

- Do the exercises prescribed by your doctor or therapist.

Mouth – Dryness, Foamy Saliva, Sores (See Nutrition for Changes in Taste)

Dryness - Dry mouth or "cotton mouth" is an excessive or abnormal dryness of the mouth related to a decrease in the quality or quantity of saliva. Dry mouth can be caused by either chemotherapy or radiation exposure to the salivary glands. Your tongue and cheeks may stick together, it may become difficult to chew and swallow foods, and your saliva may be thick and ropey. Many medicines can cause dry mouth. These include over-the-counter allergy/cough/cold/flu medicines, prescription medicines (such as those that treat anxiety and depression), pain medications, and some anti-nausea and high blood pressure medications. Dehydration can also cause dry mouth.

155

Tips for dealing with dry mouth:

- Try using an over-the-counter saliva substitute (ask your pharmacist for suggestions).
- Drink liquids between bites when eating to moisten foods and ease swallowing.
- Always carry a water bottle with you, and drink often.
- Try sucking on ice chips or hard candy.
- Try chewing sugarless gum.
- Avoid using commercial mouthwashes that contain alcohol, including lemon-glycerin swabs. These may cause increased drying and irritation to your mucosa. Instead, try mouthwashes like Biotene® or Act®.
- Add liquids to solid foods to make them more tolerable (gravies, melted butter, yogurt or mayonnaise).
- Avoid dry, sticky foods such as peanut butter, citrus fruit juice, and spicy foods, like salsa.
- Avoid alcohol and tobacco products.
- Ask your doctor for a prescription of Salegen®.

Foamy saliva – Terri - If you experience foamy saliva, try drinking Hawaiian Punch®.

Mouth Sores - These can be very painful so it is ideal to prevent them if possible. Some suggestions for dealing with mouth sores:

- Use a prescription liquid called Magic Mouthwash; this is a compound made in the pharmacy for the relief of burning mouth sores. When swished throughout the mouth, it coats the mucosa and numbs it from pain. It can be swallowed if sores are present in the throat, or it can be applied with a cotton swab to specific areas.

- Suck on ice chips when taking chemotherapy; it decreases blood flow to the cells in the mouth. **Sucking ice can help prevent mouth sores.**

- Stay away from acid-based, carbonated and caffeinated beverages.

- Eat bland, soft foods that do not require much chewing like Jell-O®, rice, soups, broth, grits, plain pasta, mashed or baked potatoes, frozen ices and ice cream.

- Avoid spicy, peppery or acidic foods.

- Try over-the-counter aids like Orabase®, Benzodent® (denture paste with 20% benzocaine), Zilactin-B®, Oragel® or Abreva®.

- Rinse your mouth after meals and at bedtime with warm salt water or baking soda and water. Another helpful rinse is a solution of equal parts of Xylocaine® viscous solution, Zovirax® (alcohol-free), and Maalox®, or Mylanta®. (If sores have developed in your throat, you can swallow a small amount for relief.) Carafate® tablets dissolved in water coats the sores and relieves pain and allows you to eat or drink.

- Use a straw for drinking liquids.

- Use unwaxed dental floss (floss only if platelet count is adequate).

- Buy a soft bristle or baby toothbrush. Cotton swabs are also effective for cleaning teeth.

- Try Vitamin E oil, Abreva® or Ulcerease® to help heal mouth sores.

Nails - Many patients who undergo chemotherapy are surprised to learn that their nails become brittle or discolored, crack easily, or even fall off completely. Fingernails are more likely to be affected than toenails due to a more rapid growth pattern. After chemotherapy begins, some people experience changes in their nail beds such as discoloration, clubbing or lifting of the nail away from the nail bed. If you lose a nail, it can take six months or longer for it to re-grow. These nail changes are especially common with chemotherapies such as Taxotere®, Taxol®, Etoposide®, and 5-FU (Fluorouracil®). Some tips for nail care:

- While receiving treatment or immediately following, submerge hands/feet in ice water to help prevent nail loss.
- Try using a product from your beauty supply store called Nail Life® that will keep your nails from deteriorating. You can also use tea tree oil on the nail beds if your nails have fallen off already.
- Do not use alcohol-based nail polish remover because the alcohol can dry the cuticle, which makes it more prone to injury and infection.
- Avoid professional manicures because the risk of infection from non-sterile instruments is too great.
- Avoid the use of artificial nails during treatment, as you are at increased risk for fungal infection.

- Wear light, cotton gloves when gardening or doing outdoor work and rubber or latex gloves when washing dishes to avoid injury to the nail bed or cuticle.

- Do not bite your nails, hangnails or cuticles. Gently trim nails and cuticles instead. Keep nails short.

- Massage a thick moisturizing cream into the nail and nail bed three to five times per week to promote healthy cuticles and encourage re-growth. Light cotton gloves at bedtime after putting lotion on can help promote moisturizing the cuticle.

- Nails that are lifting off the nail bed can be difficult to manage. Keep your nails neatly filed to keep them from catching on fabric and other items, which can cause the nail to break or tear.

- After your nails have fallen off, Band-Aid® makes an excellent gel strip, called Advanced Healing®, that protects your nail pads and promotes faster healing by sealing out water, dirt and bacteria that can cause infection.

- After heavy doses of chemo and the loss of a nail, you may experience an ingrown condition as the nail regenerates. It is important that you do not let this infection get out of control. See a wound care specialist to correct the ingrown nail and ask him/her for tips to help maintain proper growth of your nails.

- When the cuticles and nail area get dry and cracked from dehydration due to treatments, try using Nexcare® pain-free paint-on finger crack applications (similar to tissue glue).

159

If you are getting a targeted therapy, you may experience nail changes that will indicate redness and inflammation on the sides of your nails, which may become very tender and painful. A common side effect from the newer targeted therapies is (paronychia) an infection that develops along the edge of a fingernail or toenail. You should pay close attention to nail problems so that they do not lead to a severe infection. Try following these suggestions:

- Soaking nails in warm salt water with a one-part vinegar to five-part water or an antiseptic solution, several times a day is effective and try cushioning affected areas
- Apply prescription Bactroban® cream to nail area
- Topical Corticosteriods® cream
- Liquid bandages (Nexcare® cracked finger, tissue glue, etc.)
- If infection persists, call your doctor for an oral antibiotic.

Nausea (See also Vomiting) - It is easier to prevent nausea than to try to get control of it after it has already begun. There are many effective nausea medications that your doctor can prescribe for you. Some may work better than others and some may work initially but lose their effectiveness after a while. Common nausea prescriptions include Compazine®, Phenergan®, Zofran®, Ativan®, Emend®, Aloxi®, etc. Do not mix medications without a discussion with your medical team.

Terri – There has been much controversy over the use of medicinal marijuana and most cancer-help-books do not address the potential benefits. The fact remains that, for some, it provides faster nausea relief than any prescribed drug available.

The obvious downside is the inhalation of smoke into your lungs. It is illegal in most states even for medicinal purposes, so you must use your discretion with its purchase and use during treatment. In my experience, it is non-habit forming and has been a "saving grace" on many occasions when conventional pharmaceuticals have not been effective.

Unless you have specifically been told not to eat, you will probably feel better having a little something in your stomach prior to a treatment. It is important to remember to start taking your nausea medication several hours before your treatment. In some cases you may be required to start taking it the night before. Some suggestions to help diminish nausea symptoms:

- Drink ginger ale, or other carbonated drinks.
- Use fresh ginger in your foods.
- Some people report that smelling fresh newspaper can reduce nausea!
- Try drinking kraut juice (from sauerkraut, which can be purchased at a health food store).
- Nibble on soda crackers or dry toast.
- Eat dry foods such as boxed cereal, Melba® toast and cookies.
- Rather than eating two or three large meals a day, eat small, frequent, snack-size meals.
- Avoid eating greasy, fried or spicy food; instead eat bland, cold food. Bake or broil instead of frying.
- Eat salty foods like pretzels and unbuttered popcorn.

- Try sherbet and sorbet, which are light on your stomach and can be refreshing.

- Don't lie flat for at least one hour after you have eaten.

- Give your food a chance to digest properly.

- Use a cool towel on your forehead or the back of your neck.

- Try deep breathing and relaxation techniques.

- Try distraction therapy by watching a movie or listening to music.

Neuropathy (See also Hand and Foot Syndrome) - Neuropathy is also known as peripheral neuropathy and includes symptoms of tingling, numbness, burning sensations or just plain pain. It is important to let your doctor know when you begin to feel numbness and tingling (pins and needles) in your fingers and toes. You chemo dosage may be adjusted to help slow the progress of the neuropathy. The duration of neuropathy will be determined by what medications or chemotherapies were prescribed, how much you were given and how long you received them.

- If burning occurs, try immersing your feet/hands in ice water or apply cool packs.

- Try using bags of frozen peas or corn, etc. as ice packs because they conform to your feet.

- Try Vitamin B6 daily - ask doctor about dosage.

- Neuropathy from certain chemotherapy treatments can be complicated by cold sensations and you must avoid cold foods, cold air, and any contact with cold. Wear cotton gloves.

162

- Get hand and foot massages.

Nose - Like mouth sores, nose sores can be painful and can bleed easily. Try using a nasal emollient to keep your nose tissues moist in order to prevent sores. Your doctor can recommend a treatment of relief.

Terri - I have used magic mouthwash for nose sores on occasion for pain relief (applied with Q-tip). Also try Neosporin® to help heal nose sores (see Mouth sores, this chapter).

Nutrition/Diet

Be aware that each side effect may have different nutritional requirements.

Loss of Appetite or poor appetite is one of the most common side effects of chemo treatments. It may be caused by the treatment itself, depression, digestive problems, or by perceived changes in food's taste or smell. For some people loss of appetite occurs for a day or two, while for others it is an ongoing problem. Following are some suggestions to help improve your appetite:

- Start your day off by eating your largest meal for breakfast when you are hungrier.
- Eat small, frequent meals throughout the day or have a snack every couple of hours. Good snacks to try are cheese or peanut butter crackers, nuts, grated cheese, muffins, ice cream, raisins or other fruit packs, and pudding.
- Keep snacks with you when you go out so you can always have something available when you are hungry.
- Try to make your eating environment more pleasant by playing some quiet music or lighting candles.

- Eat with family or friends and try some new recipes.

- Serve meals on pretty plates to enhance your eating experience.

- Put small amounts of food on big plates to encourage yourself to finish and it will be less overwhelming.

- Extra fluid at mealtime may fill up your stomach and not allow you to finish your meals. Try to drink most of your liquids between mealtimes.

- If you don't have the time or energy for cooking, use commercial baby food to add extra protein to soups.

- Eat your meals slowly, chew food well and breathe and relax after each bite to help with digestion.

- Avoid foods with strong odors that may cause nausea.

- Avoid spicy foods that can upset your stomach.

- Avoid fried or greasy foods that might be difficult to digest or might cause acid reflux (see Indigestion). Keep away from foods that produce gas such as beans, Brussels sprouts, broccoli, cabbage, cucumbers and carbonated drinks.

- If the smell of food cooking ruins your appetite, stay out of the kitchen and ask your family or friends to cook.

- Buy a variety of foods that are easy to cook and consider making extra portions to freeze for later use when you may not feel like cooking. Remember, your body is going through many changes, so what tastes good to you now may vary from day-to-day. It's best not to stock up on one particular food.

164

- Experiment with what is most appealing to you and recognize that you may also become sensitive to food temperatures.

- Doing light exercise, a half-hour before mealtime, can help to increase your appetite. If you can, try to eat something just before you go to bed.

- If liquids have become your only source of nutrition, choose those that are high in calories. Drink supplemental beverages such as Boost® or Ensure® to help you get your basic nourishment. Most people find these more appealing if they are cold or poured over ice. Adding ingredients such as yogurt, fresh fruit, milk and tofu to instant breakfast mixes provides high calorie content, protein and vitamins. Be creative: make your own smoothie. Things like soup, juice and ice cream can give you important calories and nutrients. If you have trouble drinking enough fluid, try sucking on Popsicles® or crushed ice cubes.

You may notice weight loss if your appetite has decreased. Some foods to include in your diet to help you if you want to gain weight are: cottage cheese, ice cream, peanut butter, cream soups, wheat germ, milk (you can add one cup of nonfat dry milk to every quart of whole milk), yogurt (frozen), butter, granola, juice, pizza, eggs, cream, sour cream, mayonnaise, honey, jelly and jam, sugar, gravy, dried fruits, gelatin (Jell-O® with sugar), and bread products.

- If your doctor does not restrict alcohol and you can tolerate it, you might try a glass of wine, beer or a cocktail to increase your appetite. If alcohol disagrees with you, try a glass of orange or vegetable juice before the meal.

Change in Taste - During your treatment your sense of taste can change. Your favorite foods may become very unappealing, at least temporarily. Some foods may taste metallic or bitter while others may taste bland. Oral infections (like thrush) and certain medications can also change your sense of taste.

Some tips to help when you experience taste changes:

- Choose foods to eat that look and smell good to you.

- Remember that drinking more fluids helps to flush out the chemotherapy toxins in your body and can help food to taste better.

- Use plastic knives and forks to help offset the metallic taste of food.

- Try eating tart foods, which can sometimes mask a metallic taste. Try orange, cranberry, pineapple juices or lemonade.

- During treatment, try using the oil from a lemon peel, rubbed into your nostrils, to mask the metallic taste.

- Try sugar free-mints, sour candies, gum or ice to help mask the bitter or metallic taste.

- Rinse your mouth before you eat with a mixture of one teaspoonful of hydrogen peroxide or baking soda in a glass of distilled water; do not swallow.

- Use a toothbrush with soft bristles.

- Flavored toothpaste to clean your teeth and tongue can help improve the taste of food before you eat.

- Try mild meats such as chicken and turkey and mild-tasting fish.

- Marinate meats in sweet juices, wines, salad dressings, barbeque sauce or sweet and sour sauces.

- Use seasonings like oregano, sweet basil and rosemary on your food.

- Eat cold food, such as sherbet, fruit ice, frozen yogurt, or ice cream to numb your taste buds.

- Try different textures of food to make eating more interesting.

- Eat foods chilled or at room temperature (usually more tolerable than warm or hot foods). Chicken salad, egg salad or fruit salad are often easier to eat.

- Try foods with ginger like ginger ale, ginger snaps, or use recipes including ginger.

- Avoid tobacco products.

Excess Weight Gain - Sometimes weight gain is a problem due to certain medications, hormone or chemotherapy regimens. It can also be the result of increased appetite and eating higher calorie foods. Stress can be a contributing factor in weight gain. You could also be retaining water; your doctor might be able to help you deal with this by restricting salt or by prescribing a medicine to help you get rid of excess fluid.

Terri - Some steroids will cause you to gain weight even when you don't increase your normal intake of food. From experience, they can make you feel like you cannot fulfill the ravenous craving for food. If you are aware of this beforehand, it can

167

help you to deal with the enormous food desires that are a side effect of the drug.

Some tips to help cope with excessive weight gain:

- Remember that if you can safely exercise on a regular basis, this will always help to keep down excess body weight. For some, exercise may not be part of your daily routine but remember that staying active is very important to your overall health and recovery. Walk around your house or outside for a few minutes every day. Your normal activity level may diminish somewhat, but try to get out of bed every day and do as much activity as you can do comfortably.

- Avoid high fat, high calorie snacks such as chips, cookies, candy and ice cream.

- Try eating low fat/low calorie snacks like popcorn (air popped), graham crackers, and fresh fruit.

- Use low fat salad dressings, mayonnaise, milk, cheese and other products.

- Have fewer baked goods such as muffins, bagels, and cakes while increasing your fruit and vegetable intake.

- Eat very lean cuts of meat like chicken, turkey and fish.

Healthy Eating and Its Effects on Your Immune System - A healthy immune system is the foundation of excellent general health. There are foods that are considered carcinogenic and will directly affect your immune system. Some of them are black pepper, button mushrooms (the common cultivated variety; instead use shitake or maitake mushrooms), and peanuts and peanut products, which all contain natural carcinogens (try

168

almond or cashew butter for a healthier snack). Celery and raw legumes sprouts (alfalfa sprouts in particular) contain natural toxins that harm the immune system. In addition, heavily salted and smoked foods can be carcinogenic when consumed regularly, as are barbecued meats or any animal foods cooked until the surface is blackened. (If you have to eat these, cut away the blackened outer portion.) Reduce or eliminate cured meats-ones that look red because they have been treated with nitrate preservatives. Stop drinking chlorinated tap water and buy bottled water or filters. Avoid artificially colored foods and all artificial sweeteners, including processed sugar and flour. Eat high-fiber, whole grain products instead of refined ones. Eat plenty of fresh organic fruits and vegetables (at least six servings daily). Some important foods and their positive potential benefits include:

- Broccoli, cabbage and Brussels sprouts=can give you chemo-protective benefits
- Tomatoes = lycopene (has been found in animal studies to prevent tumor growth and decrease existing tumors)
- Citrus fruits = limonene (Vitamin C)
- Blueberries, raspberries, grapes and apples = ellagic acid (potent cancer fighter)
- All yellow and orange fruits and vegetables (also green leafy veggies) = carotenoids contain Vitamin A that may help prevent many kinds of cancer
- Soybeans = isoflavones (unusual compounds that may offer significant protection against cancer)

169

- Wild salmon and northern water fish = omega-3 fatty acids (flaxseed is an alternative to fish for omega 3's)
- Take one tablespoonful of flaxseed oil daily (do not use it in cooking)
- Garlic (potent antibiotic) and ginger (nausea and motion sickness, counters inflammation) whenever eaten raw or used in foods can have anti-tumor effects
- Use extra virgin olive oil (dark green) or expeller pressed oil in place of any processed vegetable oil (do not use any oil if it is rancid)
- Almonds and walnuts = a valuable source of omega-3 fatty acids (do not eat any nuts if rancid)
- Green tea = cancer preventive effects (drink at least one cup three times a day).

Start reading your food labels -- the food that you eat can have a direct impact on your immune system, either to hurt or to heal it.

Clear Liquid Diet

Beef or chicken broth (try Better Than Bouillon), Jell-O®, soft drinks (ginger ale, Sprite®, 7-Up®, etc.), tea, and Popsicles®

Non-Dairy Diet or Bland, Soft Diet

Soft eggs (without butter), soups, Jell-O®, pasta, soft vegetables (mashed or pureed), potatoes (mashed without milk), Ensure®, gravy (without milk), grits, applesauce, oatmeal, tea, coffee and juices (avoid caffeine if possible).

Pain, *Real and Phantom*

Real - With the resources that are available today, no one should have to experience excessive pain. **Early treatment of pain is**

almost always more effective than waiting until the pain is severe or unbearable. Under-treated and untreated pain can lead to unnecessary suffering and despair. Many different things can cause Cancer pain. You don't have to know where it's coming from to get relief, but knowing could help you feel more in control.

How to Evaluate and Describe your Own Pain The most important thing that you can do to relieve your pain is to tell your doctor or nurse about it right away. It is a good idea for you or one of your family members to keep a daily record of your pain so that you can accurately describe it to your medical team. These are some questions that you can answer to help your doctor determine your level of pain and develop a treatment plan:

- Where is your pain located? (Think of the places you feel pain.)

- How would you describe your pain? Words like "discomfort" or "hurt" don't really give your doctor accurate information. It's important to be more precise. Is it sharp? Shooting? Burning? Do you experience numbness? Does it feel different at different times? Other words you might use to describe your pain: aching, pounding, prickly, tight, deep, stabbing, pinching, dull, tender, throbbing, like a shocking pain, tingling, radiating, fullness, feeling pressure or heaviness.

- When does it hurt? When does it start? When is it better or worse? Does it wake you up at night? Does it hurt when

171

you move, when you eat, or when you are in a certain position?

- How severe is your pain? On a scale of 0 to 10, where 0 is no pain at all and 10 is the worst pain you can imagine, how would you rate your pain? (Try to be accurate.)

- What are you doing to control the pain, and is it helping? You may have found some ways to help yourself, such as taking over-the-counter medicine, using a heating pad or a cold pack. Using the same 10-point scale as above, compare your pain score from before you do what helps to about an hour afterwards.

- How does your pain affect your everyday life? Have you stopped doing certain activities like walking, climbing stairs or working? Does your pain make it difficult for you to concentrate? Do you isolate yourself from others because you are in pain? Helping your doctor or nurse understand how the pain limits your activities and affects the quality of your life will help in setting goals for dealing with your pain.

Surgery, radiation and chemotherapy can lessen and control pain caused by tumors because they can remove or reduce the size of the tumor and the source of the problem. Pain medications are also used to control pain from cancer.

Types of Pain and Pain Medicines

Mild Pain - When mild pain is present, acetaminophen (Tylenol®) and other nonsteroidal anti-inflammatory medications (NSAIDS) are recommended. These include aspirin and ibuprofen (Motrin® and Advil®), and most are available without a prescription. NSAIDS, used alone, have a limit to their pain-relieving effect; so don't take a higher dose than specified. Aspirin, although an excellent pain reliever, is not often given to people receiving radiation or chemotherapy because it acts as a blood thinner.

Moderate to severe pain - For this level of pain you may need an opioid, which requires a prescription. Morphine, Fentanyl®, hydromorphone, Oxycodone® and codeine are all opioids. They can be taken by mouth (pill or liquid), through a patch on the body, in suppository form, or by injection. Your doctor or pain team may need to increase the dose of these medications in order to relieve your pain. Sometimes your doctor may prescribe nonopioids along with opioids for this kind of pain. Many people resist taking potentially helpful medications such as morphine because they fear drug addition. While addiction is possible with long-term use of opioids, it is more important to have adequate pain control.

Pain from Swelling - This pain is often treated with steroids. Examples of steroids include Prednisone® and Decadron®. Prescriptions are necessary for these medications. It is important to follow directions carefully when taking these medications. Do not stop taking these medications suddenly without letting your doctor know. Steroids need to be tapered (decreased) slowly over time.

Nerve Pain - Antidepressants may be prescribed for you to relieve symptoms such as the burning and tingling that occurs from nerve pain. Taking antidepressants does not mean you are depressed, unable to cope or crazy. Amitriptyline® and Imapramine® are examples of antidepressants, but there are many others.

Managing Side Effects from Pain Medication - Like most medications, pain medications have side effects. It is best to know what they are before you start taking them, so you will be prepared and feel less anxious. It is also important to know that many of the side effects can be treated to help maintain your quality of life. The most common side effects of pain medicines are constipation, nausea and vomiting, and drowsiness. Other milder side effects include dizziness, slowed breathing, dry mouth, itchy skin, confusion and fluid retention. If you experience any of these side effects, report them to your doctor because they can be treated. Either the dosage can be changed, or another method of pain relief can be tried.

Reducing Pain Without Drugs - There are many ways to help relieve pain without drugs. Relaxation, meditation, distraction therapy, guided imagery, visualization, skin stimulation (such as massages, heating pads or ice packs), exercise and support groups are all very effective and simple techniques used to help reduce pain levels. See PART V, CHAPTERS NINE and TEN for alternative methods of pain relief.

Phantom - Phantom sensation is sometimes experienced after having a part of your body surgically removed. It is often described as resembling a tingling sensation. Severe discomfort or pain near the area is referred to as phantom pain. Those who experience this find, that in most cases, it decreases with time.

End of Life (Palliative) Care: Pain and Symptom Management

Palliative care is prevention and relief of pain offered to people who are terminally ill. This specific care pays attention to the physical, emotional, spiritual and practical needs of patients and those caring for them. Palliative care regards dying as a normal process and provides relief from pain and other distressing symptoms. It helps contribute to what one might consider a "good" death, a death free from avoidable suffering and stress for patients and their caregivers.

Hospice (or hospice care) is the setting where people who are terminally ill receive palliative care. Hospice care can take place either in your home or in a home-like facility. The goals of hospice care are to control pain, provide palliative care, and preserve the highest possible quality of life for as long as life remains. Discussing end of life issues is never easy. Most people have not learned how to talk realistically and comfortably about dying. The resulting fear and misinformation can lead to the mistaken belief that pain and misery at death are unavoidable. It is possible to reduce end-of-life pain and suffering, but some patients and their families don't realize all their options. Our society is learning that the dying phase can still be an important, valuable time in a person's life. Being aware of, and asking for, hospice and palliative care services may be helpful for patients and caregivers. Some things to remember are the following:

- A person with cancer and those who care about them might have a difficult time accepting or understanding a prognosis that is terminal. Talking about these issues can be uncomfortable and complicate decision making. A social worker or other health care professional can help guide you through the processes that lie ahead.

- If there is no further treatment available, people often think that that there is nothing left that can be done. On the contrary, much can be done for someone who is terminally ill. The type of care given now has a different focus, and there are many options.

- Many end of life concerns come from fear of either over-treatment (too much aggressive care) or abandonment (getting no care). It is best to acknowledge these fears and work with the healthcare team to find an acceptable balance.

- Many times patients, families or caregivers think it is too soon to start hospice care and wait until death is very near. Bringing hospice professionals in at the last minute makes it difficult for them to provide the care that is needed. A suggested approach is to arrange preliminary home meetings and counseling with hospice and/or other health professionals who can provide for the care of your loved one. Building a support network before a crisis helps to ease additional stress.

Rash – A common side effect from the newer targeted therapies is a body rash. It may start on your face as a raised rash and will move to other areas of your body as you continue using the antibody. It may begin to subside after using the antibody over a period of time. Some things to help relieve the side effects of a rash are:

- Moisturize your body with heavy moisturizers or massage oils several times a day.

- Do not pop or squeeze pustules.

- Take only lukewarm showers; do not sit in hot bath water.

- Limit sun exposure; wear a hat or UV clothing.

- Use topical prescription creams, such as metronidazole or Elidel®.

- Avoid creams containing vitamin A because they can aggravate skin rashes.

- Stay hydrated by drinking recommended daily fluids.

- If itching occurs, ask for a prescription of Atarax®; also see section on Itching, this chapter.

- Try Neutrogena T-Gel® shampoo as soap for your whole body.

Sex - Your sexual feelings are not a usual part of the treatment plan you discuss with your oncologist. Although talking about sex may seem "taboo" because of its intimate nature, sexuality is an important part of everyone's life. Since cancer affects all aspects of your life, that would include your sexual feelings as well. It is common during the course of your chemotherapy to have times when you lose the desire to have sex, or even the ability to have sexual activity in the way you did before your disease. Factors that may contribute to this loss are fatigue; weight changes; nausea; depression; anxiety; pain; and self-consciousness or low self-esteem resulting from loss of hair or removal of a body part.

For women there may be pain or difficulty in having intercourse due to a narrowing of the vagina or vaginal dryness, resulting from radiation, chemotherapy or surgery. Sometimes chemotherapy, surgery or pelvic radiation can cause premature menopause. Loss of estrogen can trigger hot flashes and vaginal atrophy, in which the vagina becomes tight and dry (see Hot Flashes, this section). Some women can take replacement hormones to help with these problems; however, women with breast or uterine cancer usually cannot take estrogen or estrogen supplements.

Terri – Recently, a vaginal insert called Vagifem® was released for women who absolutely cannot allow miniscule amounts of estrogen into their bloodstream. I am estrogen receptor positive and have been using this pill with excellent results. Vaginal estrogen may be an option, but get the prescription approved by your oncologist before using.

If intercourse is still an option for you but is more difficult due to dryness, there are several good non-prescription vaginal lubricants that can help ease this difficulty. These include: Replens®, K-Y Jelly®, and Astroglide® *Terri - Astroglide® is the preferred lubricant.* A woman having chemotherapy, or the female partner of a man having chemotherapy, can get pregnant during treatment. It is very important to avoid pregnancy during chemotherapy and for a while afterwards in case the drugs affect the baby. Use reliable contraception. If you are a woman being treated, and have been on the contraceptive pill, ask your doctor whether it is all right for you to continue. It is also a good idea to use a condom.

For men - Besides lowered sex drive, cancer treatments may cause difficulty in getting and maintaining an erection and inability to ejaculate. Treatments for these difficulties can include drug therapy such as Viagra®, Cialis®, injections, vacuum pumps, or even penile implants. Sometimes no treatment is needed since normal erectile function may return after treatment has ended. You may want to consider banking your sperm before receiving your first chemo treatment.

If sexual intimacy has been a vital part of your life, you may want to continue to be sexually active even while dealing with your disease. Some expected changes will occur but you can still achieve sexual intimacy during this time. It is good to remember that your mind is the true source of your sexuality. Talking with your partner openly is the best way to start. Whatever gives both of you physical pleasure and/or comfort together is normal for you. Sexual expressions are not limited to intercourse. Consider kissing, body massage, self-stimulation and oral sex as alternatives. Having a warm, caring, loving body lying next to you is immensely satisfying, and gentle stroking and hugging are good for both body and soul. They help you emotionally and increase your sense of well-being. There is more to sex, love and affection than simple intercourse.

Shingles (See also Itching) - Shingles is an infection caused by the nerve virus that causes chicken pox. It only occurs in people who have had chicken pox and is caused by a weakened immune system. When your body fights off chicken pox, it doesn't get rid of the virus; instead it goes dormant in your nervous system. The first sign of shingles is usually a tingly, itchy feeling or a stabbing pain on the skin. After a few days a rash appears as raised dots on your body or face (similar to chicken pox). It then develops into small, fluid-filled blisters that dry and crust. Associated pain can range from mild to severe. At the first sign of shingles, you should notify your doctor immediately. There are prescription medications available to relieve the pain and itching. Helpful medications include: Acyclovir®, steroids (Prednisone®), nerve blocks, narcotics and anti-depressants such as Elavil®. Shingles unrecognized or untreated can become a severe medical problem. The earlier it is treated the better. See Itching in this section for more helpful hints for relief.

Skin - Your skin is the largest organ in your body and functions like a sponge. Everything that you put on your skin is absorbed into your tissue and bloodstream. Try using more natural products with fewer chemicals from health food stores or the internet. Start reading labels and learn about what you are putting on your body. While undergoing chemo, your body can react differently to products that you've used for years.

Things you can do to protect your skin:

- Eat more protein to promote faster skin healing.
- Drink eight 8-ounce glasses of water daily.
- Use electric shavers instead of razors.
- Bathe and shower with warm, not hot water, once a day.

- Use gentle soap with no perfumes, like Castile, glycerin, Dove®, Cetaphil® or Ivory®.
- Don't scrub the skin and pat dry gently.
- Avoid extremes in temperature (like ice packs or heating pads on the skin).
- Don't use cologne or perfume, which can dry skin.
- Use gentle moisturizers such as Cetaphil®, Nexcare Advanced Healing® and Aveeno®.
- If you develop any sores try using Wounded Warrior®, a natural astringent.
- Don't pop blisters.

To protect sensitive skin against sunburn:

- Use a sun block of SPF 30+.
- Wear a wide-brimmed hat.
- Limit sun exposure to early morning and early evening.
- Cover skin with long sleeves and pants or UV clothing.

A common side effect of some chemotherapies is a change in skin pigments. Hyperpigmentation is a darkening of the skin, which may occur under your nails, around your mouth, on the palms of your hands and soles of your feet, along the veins used for chemo, and on your face and body generally. A fade cream with the ingredient hydraquinone (such as Esoterica®) can be found at your cosmetic counter or your pharmacy and can help to lessen the dark spots. After you have finished your chemotherapy your pigmentation should return to normal.

Skin care during radiation therapy

You will need to be very gentle with the skin in the treated area. The majority of skin reactions to radiation will go away in a few weeks after treatment has been completed. In some cases, your skin may remain slightly darker than before and may be more sensitive to the sun. The following suggestions may be helpful when caring for your skin during radiation:

- Apply 100% aloe vera cream or the gel inside of an aloe leaf from an aloe plant to the affected area.
- When you wash use only lukewarm water and mild soap, and pat dry. Do not rub, scrub, or scratch the skin in the treated area.
- Do not wear tight clothing over the radiated area.
- Do not apply any skin lotions within two hours of a treatment.
- Avoid any powders, creams, perfumes, deodorants, body oils, ointments, lotions, or home remedies in the treated area unless approved by your doctor or nurse.
- Avoid exposure to the sun or wear protective clothing until your doctor clears you.

Skin care during targeted therapies

- Moisturize your body with heavy moisturizers or massage oils several times a day. Try Nexcare Advanced Healing®.
- Do not pop or squeeze pustules.
- Take only lukewarm showers; do not sit in hot bath water.
- Use topical prescription creams, such as metronidazole or Elidel®.

- Drink eight 8-ounce glasses of water daily.

- If itching occurs, ask for a prescription of Atarax®, also see section on Itching, this chapter.

- Use gentle soap with no perfumes, like castile, glycerin, Dove®, Ivory® or Cetaphyl®.

- Don't scrub the skin; pat dry gently or use a hair dryer.

- Try to use all natural products; rash will make your skin extra sensitive, especially on your face.

To protect sensitive skin against sunburn:

- Use a sun block of SPF 30+.

- Wear a wide-brimmed hat and protective clothing.

Sleeplessness (Sleep Deprivation) - Sleeplessness or insomnia can be a very frustrating experience. Not being able to fall asleep naturally can be attributed to many factors during chemotherapy, but stress is the main one. Certain steroids also can leave you looking at the ceiling and counting sheep.

Some tips to help you sleep:

- Before you go to bed, do things that will help you relax such as: ✔ read or listen to soothing music ✔ take a warm bath. ✔ make the bedroom quiet and cool.

- Avoid drinking caffeinated drinks and avoid tobacco since nicotine is a stimulant.

- Take medications early in the day if possible.

- Stop drinking fluids after eight p.m. to prevent having to get up to urinate in the night.

- Establish a sleep routine by going to bed at the same time each night.

- Use your bed for sleeping only (not reading, working, watching TV, etc.).

- Use a white noise machine or fan to filter disturbing noise.

- There are prescription sleep medications (like Ambien®) that allow you to wake up feeling non-drowsy. Contact your doctor if you feel you need a sleep aid.

Swelling (Also call edema) - Chemotherapy can cause the body to retain fluid. Symptoms may include swelling or puffiness in the face, hands, feet or abdomen. In particular, Adriamyacin® can sometimes cause swelling and is indicative of a more serious condition called congestive heart failure. Contact your doctor immediately if you think you may be having this side effect while taking this drug. What you can do to help:

- Limit or avoid table salt and salty foods.

- Exercise as much as possible; this aids circulation.

- Don't sit for long periods of time.

- When resting, try to elevate your legs and feet.

- When traveling by air, get up several times during the flight and walk through the aisle to prevent swelling and clotting.

Call your doctor if you notice any of the above symptoms. Medications may be recommended to get rid of the excess fluid.

Teeth - Have any necessary dental work completed before you begin your treatment. The National Cancer Institute recommends that you give yourself time to heal from any dental work by scheduling a dental check-up at least two to four weeks before starting chemo or radiation. Be sure to tell your dentist that you will be undergoing treatment.

Good dental tips:

- Take especially good care of your teeth and gums.
- Buy a new toothbrush after each monthly cycle of chemotherapy. (This will ensure that your toothbrush is clean and free of any bacterial/chemical residue.)
- If you wear dentures, clean them after each meal.
- Brush your teeth with gentle strokes and use care when flossing using unwaxed dental floss. If bleeding occurs, do not panic but do stop flossing for a few days. If this persists or you are concerned about it, let your doctor know.

Throat - Dysphagia means difficulty with chewing or swallowing food or liquid. Swallowing is a reflex that people do not actively control. A swollen or sore throat, cancer of the throat or larynx, or dry mouth can cause swallowing to be difficult. The following are helpful guidelines for swallowing:

- Sit in an upright position (as near 90 degrees as possible) whenever eating or drinking.
- Cut food into small bites -- only one half to one teaspoonful at a time.
- Eat slowly and chew thoroughly.
- Avoid talking while eating.
- Eat in a relaxed atmosphere with no distractions.
- Avoid solid and hard-to-swallow foods.
- Try high calorie liquids, like Ensure®, etc., and drink them through a straw.

- Try using a prescription of Magic Mouthwash, which is safe to swallow, for sores in your throat. It coats the mucosa and numbs it from pain.

- If you have difficulty swallowing pills, try coating them in butter.

Urine – A burning sensation while urinating is a common side effect of chemo and is caused by the toxicity of the chemical running through your body. This condition is called cystitis and can also occur as a result of radiation. It is very important to drink plenty of fluids, especially water or cranberry juice. Contact your doctor immediately if the burning persists so that a relief medication can be prescribed and to make sure that you don't have a urinary tract infection. Remember to keep your genital area very clean to prevent infection. (For women, after a bowel movement, wipe from front to back so that you don't get bacteria into your vagina.)

Vomiting (See also Nausea) - Vomiting can be brought on by chemotherapy, emotional stress, pain, strong odors, motion changes, and indigestion. It can be controlled by antiemetic medication. If you are vomiting continuously, it is important to remember that you can easily become dehydrated and should let your doctor know your condition. Some tips to help when vomiting:

- Avoid eating or drinking until vomiting has stopped. Once you have vomiting under control, you may begin to take small amounts of clear liquids.

- o Start with one teaspoonful of water, ice chips or bouillon every ten minutes.

- o Increase the amount gradually to one tablespoonful every 20 minutes, and then try two tablespoonfuls every 30 minutes.

- o When you can keep clear liquids down, try a full liquid diet (ice, Jell-O®, broth, Popsicles®, clear juice) or a soft diet (milk, cereal, ice-cream, pudding, custard, soup).

- o Continue taking small amounts and gradually work up to returning to your regular diet.

- Drink chamomile or ginger root tea.
- Try dry toast or crackers to settle your stomach.
- Change from a sitting to a standing position slowly.
- Avoid odors from cooking foods.
- Try to keep cool and keep the air moving around you (with a fan or open window).
- Use alcohol-free mouthwash to remove any aftertaste from vomiting.

Part IV – Side Effects

PART V

Nurturing Your Inner Self

CHAPTER EIGHT

Looking and Feeling Better

Cosmetics, (See also Skin Care, Part IV)

How we see ourselves often reflects how we feel. Even though you may not feel well, putting on some make-up boosts your spirits and can make you feel better.

- Try a bronzing powder or lotion to help you maintain a healthy glow. Most cosmetics contain chemicals, and you may become sensitive to the products that you have used for years. Consider using a natural mineral powder for facial coverage, such as Bare Minerals®.

- If you've experienced tearing problems, try using waterproof mascara and liners to eliminate running of makeup.

- Eyebrows give expression to the face. If you lose your eyebrows or forget how they were shaped, you can purchase stencils (at some cosmetic counters) to use and fill them in with a pencil or powder.

The American Cancer Society offers a program called "Look Good, Feel Better" at most cancer centers, and it is free of charge. These sessions provide make-up techniques, information on the different wigs that are available and ways to wear hats, scarves and head coverings to make you feel better.

Nancy – My mother always said, "a little make-up never hurt anyone" and I think she was right. In fact, it may help, because it helps you project a healthy feeling to yourself and to others. Skin care is important while taking chemo and radiation because these treatments do affect the texture of your skin. A side effect of treatment that can be beneficial is the loss of facial hair, which can give your complexion a very flattering luminous look.

Exercise

Regular exercise is important in many ways to your overall health. Among many benefits, exercise can:

- Help keep you limber and strong
- Relieve stress and tension
- Help elevate mood
- Stimulate the process of digestion, absorption, metabolism, and elimination
- Help prevent osteoporosis
- Help you sleep better
- Stimulate the brain, helping to improve memory and attention span
- Help regulate weight
- Increase your sense of control and improves your self-esteem.

Some studies show that regular exercise might even help to prevent certain forms of cancer. Many oncologists advise their patients to stay as active as possible during treatment. If you had a regular exercise program before diagnosis and treatment, try to maintain as much of your regimen as you can; doing so will help give you increased vitality, and a sense of control and accomplishment at a time when you need it most. If you were relatively inactive before, there are still some things you can do that will be beneficial to you. In either case, what type of exercise you do will depend on several factors, including: your past and present fitness level, your type and stage of cancer, the drugs you are taking and your reaction to them. Follow the fundamental guidelines for any beginner exercise program:

- Start slowly, and build up gradually.
- Begin with a light warm-up and end with a cool-down.
- Slow down or stop if it hurts or you get too tired.

There are ordinary activities that you can do to increase your level of activity without a special program; among these are walking, cleaning, making the bed, climbing the stairs, playing with children and gardening. Even if you are confined to bed or a wheelchair, there are some things you can do to keep from getting weak and progressively more fatigued. If you have your doctor's permission and if you are physically able, try some of these exercises:

- Move your feet and wiggle your toes.
- Raise your arms above your head.
- Lift your legs.
- Shrug your shoulders.
- Do deep breathing exercises (see Breathwork, CHAPTER ELEVEN).

You need to check with your doctor before you begin any exercise program and ask if it is appropriate in your particular situation. In general, wait to exercise until at least 24 hours after having a treatment. Don't exercise if you have an irregular pulse or a resting pulse of more than 100; if you have chest pain, fever, or infection; or if you have extreme pain. Additionally, if you are exercising, stop immediately and consult your doctor if you experience any of the following symptoms: irregular heartbeats, shortness of breath or difficulty breathing, chest pains, leg cramping, dizziness or nausea.

Wigs

Try to begin shopping for a wig well before you expect your hair to start falling out. You may want to involve your hairdresser in your search for a wig. Try different colors and styles and have fun with the experience. Once you have found the right wig, wear it to your beauty shop and have your hairdresser cut it to your style. Experience in cutting wigs is helpful because it WON'T grow back. Usually most wigs are too thick and need to be thinned by an expert. Synthetic wigs are less expensive than human hair wigs and they hold their shape and shine better. Use caution around open flames or steam because heat will singe the wig. When you wear your wig, try wearing a headband or a sun-visor with it. This makes it look more natural and helps to hold it on. Most insurance companies will reimburse patients for the full cost or partial cost of a wig. You may need to obtain a pre-authorization from your insurance company; the insurance company may have only certain vendors from which they allow you to purchase a wig. Consult your policy or call your insurance company to determine what your provider covers. In order to obtain a reimbursement, you must submit a receipt and a prescription from your doctor. Your doctor will write a prescription for an "extra cranial prosthesis for chemotherapy-induced alopecia." Medicare and some insurance companies do not pay for wigs, but you should keep your receipt because it is a medical expense and may be tax deductible. If you participate in a flex plan where you work, the wig may qualify as a medical expense. Many hospitals have assistance available with wig lending through patient support programs. For help with wig purchases, see the Resource section of this book.

CHAPTER NINE

Living Better

Acupuncture/ Acupressure

Acupuncture is a treatment in which thin needles are inserted through the skin at specific anatomical points on the body and are manipulated by hand or electrical stimulation to control pain and relieve other health problems. The locations of these points, mapped out over 2000 years ago by the Chinese, have recently been confirmed by electromagnetic research. Traditional acupuncture is based on Chinese theories of the flow of energy (Qi) and blood (Xue) through distinct pathways (meridians) that run throughout the body. Qi is believed to regulate spiritual, emotional, mental and physical balance and to be influenced by the opposing forces in the body called yin and yang. Acupuncture is used to help balance yin and yang, to keep the normal flow of energy unblocked, and to restore health to the mind and body. It has been used very effectively to aid in pain control and to reduce nausea associated with chemotherapy. Acupuncture is a licensed and regulated healthcare treatment in about half of the United States. If you decide to have acupuncture, check your practioner's credentials.

Acupressure is a non-needle variation of acupuncture involving deep finger pressure applied to certain acupoints.

It is rooted in the traditional Chinese medicine and actually predates acupuncture.

Biofeedback

Biofeedback is method of treatment that uses monitoring devices to help you control body processes that are normally controlled automatically. Under the guidance of a therapist (one certified by the Biofeedback Certification Institute of America), you concentrate to try to change a body function like heart rate, perspiration, blood flow, muscle tension or body temperature. The therapist attaches electrodes to various points on your body. (For example, if you have headache or sleeplessness, they would be attached to your scalp.) The sensors are connected to a monitor that signals changes in these body functions by a graph, beep, buzz, a light or some other method that can be measured. The therapist teaches you mental or physical exercises that can help you affect the function that is troubling you. By observing the monitor, you can see whether or not you are having success. Gradually, you can learn to associate successful thoughts and actions with the changes you desire in your responses. Like most mind-body therapies, biofeedback is free of side effects, but if you have a pacemaker, you should check with your doctor before using a monitor which might interfere with your device.

Healing Touch

Touch is both an effective way of healing and one of the most powerful means for giving and receiving love. Biblically, the spiritual aspect of touch is expressed as the "laying on of hands." Healing touch uses touch to affect the human energy system, specifically the energy field that surrounds the body, and the energy centers that control the flow from the energy field to the physical body. These non-invasive methods utilize the hands to clear, energize, and balance the human and environmental energy fields. Proponents of healing touch report that it can help heal wounds, relieve headaches, reduce pain, lessen anxiety, promote relaxation, and help the body to restore itself to health. The practice of healing touch rarely involves actual physical contact; instead, the therapist moves his/her hands above the patient's body. Those who have experienced it report that healing touch gives them relaxation and a sense of deep peace. To choose a healing touch practitioner, look for someone who has completed a workshop and has used the technique under the guidance of a mentor, preferably for at least a year. Nurse Healers (215-545-8079) offers a list of practitioners.

Herbal Supplements

If you take herbal supplements to help with your appetite or with any side effects of your chemotherapy and treatment, be sure to tell your doctor exactly what you are taking since these may interact with your medications. Herbs are the oldest medicines known to man, and many of today's current medications are based on plants, for example digitalis (foxglove); aspirin (white willow); and morphine (opium poppy). Because they are natural and available without prescription, many people view herbal medicines as safe. Unfortunately, not all herbs are benign, and some can even be dangerous, especially used in combination with other drugs. The FDA does not regulate herbs, and the strength and ingredients may vary. Information about possible side effects and/or dangers may not be available. It's extremely important that you choose a reliable source for herbs. If used carefully, they can provide safe treatment for many ailments in the same way as over-the-counter drugs.

Here are some things that might help:

- Ask your doctor and your pharmacist about each herb.

- Try to select manufacturers you recognize.

- Choose brand labels that are natural and have amounts listed in understandable form.

- Learn as much as you can about an herb's potential toxicity and possible drug interactions before you take it. Contact http://www.consumerlab.com/ for analysis of ingredients.

Massage

Massage is the healing art that creates balance and restores the necessary sense of well-being. Anyone who has ever given or received a friendly backrub already knows something about massage therapy. It is a systematic manual application of pressure and movement to the soft tissue of the body. Massage promotes the flow of blood and lymphatic fluids, stimulates nerves, relieves tension, and loosens muscles and connective tissue. Among its many benefits, massage can:

- Promote relaxation

- Help alleviate pain

- Reduce anxiety

- Lower stress levels

- Lower blood pressure and heart rate.

In the past, massage has been considered a luxury; now it is recognized as an important technique in the integrative healing arts. There are many different types of massage available today (Swedish, deep tissue, hot stone, lymph system, deep muscle, reflexology, Reiki, Shiatsu, Thai, and trigger point). Before you receive one, make sure that you fully understand the type of massage that you will be given. Massage is not recommended if you have an infectious skin disease, a rash, an unhealed wound, varicose veins, or if you are prone to blood clots. It is recommended that you consult with your oncologist before scheduling massage therapy. If you decide to have a massage, choose a therapist who is properly qualified, preferably a member of the American Massage Therapy Association.

Music

Healing through music is an unconventional method of caring for your body. It is soothing to the soul and has been proven to relax your mind in the most tense of situations. Doctors and dentists use it in their offices to calm the nerves of patients. Businesses use it to sooth irate customers who are holding on the phone. Musicians are brought in to treatment areas to play for patients for a calming effect and to comfort the weary. From listening to Mozart to strumming a guitar, many people can benefit from music's calmative effects.

A unique method of musical healing is known as the Tibetan singing bowls. These bowls diversify the possibilities for healing with vibrations and sounds. Testimony indicates that benefits are physical, psychological and spiritual all at the same time. Music can also help to accomplish the following:

- Lower your blood pressure, heart and breathing rate
- Helps to prevent insomnia
- Relieve stress and muscle tension
- Provide relaxation.

Andrew Weil, MD, who has done much research on the healing properties of certain music, writes, "I have long been interested in healing and how to stimulate it. I know that the human body has a healing system, that it can repair and regenerate itself. I also know that the body wants to be healthy, that it wants to come back to the state of balance where all systems operate efficiently. Sound is an especially powerful influence on the human nervous system. It can harm and it can heal. Whether you are ill or injured, facing a surgical procedure, suffering an emotional hurt or simply want to maintain optimum health, music sounds can help you to heal."

No one knows exactly how music benefits the body, but one theory holds that our muscles, including the heart muscle, learn to synchronize to the beat of the music. Another theory suggests that music and sound distract the mind from focusing on pain and anxiety. An additional source of tranquility for the mind is listening to different sounds of water: raindrops falling, a babbling brook, ocean waves, or a mountain waterfall. Use the plentiful music resources available to quiet your mind, relax your body and elevate your spirit.

Nancy – Today I had an MRI on my spine. The machine makes a loud, clacking noise. As I lay there listening, I found myself making music to the clacks. I realized that everything has its own music – even an MRI machine. Birds have their own music, bugs have their music – every species of life has its own music. It's wonderful when we can resonate with the music of other things, even a machine.

Pet Therapy

Sometimes you need to tell your troubles, fears and worries to someone who just listens whenever you want to talk. Do you have a special someone with four paws and a tail (or perhaps two wings and a beak) that doesn't comment on bald heads or bruised arms? A scratch behind the ears, from a weak hand, can give both the giver and the receiver a sense of peace and comfort. One such resource may be right at your feet; if so, be sure to take advantage of the gifts it can bring you. Animals possess the wonderful ability to live in the moment, and in a special way, they are able to share with you where you are right then and there. A wet nose appearing at the edge of the bed or a soft paw batting at your arm can be a call to share the moment in the most basic way, which is simply to be together. A dog needing a walk may provide the encouragement needed to get a little exercise. Time spent at home is not time alone when there is a pet in the house. Just knowing that another living being is nearby can bring a sense of reassurance. If you are hospitalized for a period of time, you may want to inquire if your hospital has a pet therapy program; some have such a program in conjunction with their recreational therapy department.

Progressive Muscle Relaxation

This is a technique used to relax your entire body systematically by alternately tensing and relaxing individual parts of it. By tensing muscles first and then relaxing them, you become aware of how a truly relaxed muscle feels. (Sometimes you are actually tense when you think that you have relaxed, and this helps to show the difference.) Muscle relaxation can be used to help control pain and to relieve anxiety or to help achieve a calm state for meditation. Here is a short form of this exercise you might wish to try: Begin by sitting or lying down in a comfortable position in a quiet room. Close your eyes and become aware of your breathing. First focus on your right foot, and flex your toes back very hard, holding them this way for a few seconds, and then let them go completely limp. Gradually, work your way up your right leg by tensing each muscle group individually, and then relaxing it. Then do your left toes and legs. Follow this same procedure for your hips, waist, back, chest, hands, arms, shoulders, neck, scalp, and face. Raise your eyebrows, open your eyes wide, scrunch your face and lips, and then completely relax your face muscles. Then raise your arms over your head and stretch. Tense every muscle at once, and then relax. Return focus to your breathing, and rest.

Self-hypnosis

Trance is an altered state of consciousness (like daydreaming), and hypnosis is the method used to achieve it. You can be taught to get yourself into this hypnotic state so that you can control when the trance will occur. You can use it to enhance relaxation and healing. Self-hypnosis, like meditation, involves an initial period of concentration on an object. Hypnosis does not try to keep your awareness in the present; instead, you enter into a deeply relaxed, somewhat sub-conscious state of mind. Try these suggestions for self-hypnosis:

- Take a slow deep controlled breath, in through your nose and out through your mouth; hear your breath.

- Put your thumb and index finger together and take another slow deep breath.

- With the next deep breath, apply slight pressure between your two fingers; as you exhale, relax your two fingers and let your mind take you to a favorite place of soothing, peaceful surroundings.

- Continue the breath patterns while maintaining the method of relaxing with each exhalation.

- Stay there as long as you'd like for optimum benefits.

Hypnosis is a valuable aid in controlling pain and helping to relieve stress and anxiety.

Support Groups

Being active in a support group can be a great source of therapy if you take advantage of it, and there is no charge for participating. Groups are formed to offer support to patients, family members and caregivers of people with cancer. Other patients and families who have had the experience of cancer can offer valuable information and stories to help ease concerns during this time in your life. They present information, provide comfort, help to reduce anxiety, teach coping skills and help you to feel as though you are not going through this experience alone. Usually, you will be directed to a group of people who have the same type of cancer that you do or one composed of people undergoing the same type of treatment that you are. Support groups meet at different times, on different days, and for different types of cancer. They may be led by survivors of cancer, other group members, or by trained professionals. They focus on learning to manage current concerns and situations through education, behavioral training or group interaction. Ask your doctor or nurse for information about support groups.

Support Relationships

All people need support relationships in order to live full lives; but when you are dealing with cancer, those important relationships are vital to your survival. You may not be fortunate enough to be able to count on your family to support you during this or other difficult times; or you may choose not to share this crisis with your spouse or loved ones for fear of upsetting or burdening them. It might be that you are having a difficult time facing the ramifications of your cancer, or perhaps your family member or friend is struggling to cope and is unable to help you. Whatever the cause, when you can't call on your family or friends for support, you will have a greater burden to bear. Realize that there are many people who can serve as caregivers. In fact, in some cases it might be easier to tell your troubles to people whom you don't know well, people who can be more objective and who are experienced listeners. Never underestimate the power of love, even from someone whom you thought wasn't capable of dealing with a crisis. There are alternative sources for emotional support; among these are your ministers, social workers, patient volunteers, support groups, psychotherapists or family therapists. The people who support you emotionally are the ones you can lean on in times of trouble; they are special angels who are vital to helping you get through this experience. Encourage your caregiver to take time alone or just away from the cancer world for a short time. Doing this will reward you with the greatest health benefit of all – the gift of love. Remember that your role as a lover, spouse, parent, child, neighbor and/or friend, is the most powerful opportunity for connection and spiritual growth. Commit to becoming more conscious in all your relationships, especially the most intimate ones. There is a divine spark, a life-force energy, residing within each of us. By honoring that spark in your loved ones, you help them become more of who and what they are - human embodiments of Spirit. In return, they help you to do the same. Don't take your relationships for granted. Instead, cultivate wonder and gratitude for all the gifts you are able to share with your loved ones.

Visualization

Visualization is a powerful self-help tool. Most of the time visualizing is done unconsciously when we daydream. Researchers and physicians have been trying to capture these mental images to help create a heightened state of well-being.

Because of their research, thousands of people are learning to use visualization to enhance their health. Like most of the other therapies outlined in this chapter, this technique can be used to create positive change in almost any area of your life. All that is necessary is a willingness to practice and develop this as a positive habit. Visualization helps to improve and maintain health because of the ability to affect our bodies at a cellular level. Since mental images are so deeply connected to our emotions and the events in our lives, they help us to discover more effective solutions for our health and other problems. To practice a simple visualization, do the following exercises: You can sit comfortably in a chair or lie down in bed. Select a time and place when you will not be disturbed. Close your eyes and focus on your breathing. Take a few deep, unforced breaths to help yourself relax. With each inhalation, imagine a soothing, relaxing energy flowing through all areas of your body. As you exhale, visualize the cares and concerns of the day gradually disappearing. Do this for two or three minutes, allowing your breath to carry you to a place of calm relaxation. Remember a time before your diagnosis of cancer; for example, when you could run or climb stairs easily. Allow yourself to re-experience that time, using all of your senses to imagine it as it actually happened. Try to recall what you saw, tasted, smelled, heard and felt during that time. Once you have reconnected, bring it into the present as if it were happening now. Stay in that place for at least five minutes, convincing yourself that you are experiencing the desired state in the present. When you first try visualization, don't be discouraged if it seems that nothing is happening. Like anything new, seeing results takes time. Some large treatment centers offer virtual reality during chemotherapy to help distract your mind from the treatment so that you can minimize the side effects that might occur.

Yoga

Yoga is one of the most invigorating and stimulating gifts you can give to your body. It is a form of non-aerobic exercise used to help the body naturally heal and balance itself with precise posture and breathing. The most common form of yoga uses movement, breathing, exercise and meditation to help you to connect with the mind, body, and spirit. The goal is to guide you from your present state of awareness into a state of wholeness, well-being, and enlightenment. With some basic instruction, even a beginner can achieve the benefits of relieving physical and mental tension and improving concentration while maintaining a valuable fitness regimen. This is a basic outline of some yoga practices:

- You will begin by focusing on your breath, inhaling and exhaling with some warm-up exercises.
- Yoga consists of 10-12 gentle poses. Each pose is used to stimulate circulation to a certain part of the body and improve the health of muscles and internal organs.
- The movements are very slow, smooth, and controlled with each inhalation and exhalation of your breath.
- Yoga ends with a period of rest and meditation.

- You may continue yoga as long as it is helpful to you. Many people have adopted yoga and practiced it for life.
- Check with your doctor for any specific limitations.

CHAPTER TEN

Personal Resources

≋APPRECIATING TIME

Susan - Time: 12 months in a year; 7 days in a week; 24 hours in a day; 60 minutes in an hour. When all is going well in life, it is easy to take time for granted. Life gets so busy at times that we don't appreciate the special moments given to us daily. Cancer will provide you with the opportunity to re-organize your priorities. Sharing your life with people you love becomes your concern in place of material things. Slowing down allows you to focus on the person you are with and to enjoy their presence rather than being preoccupied with the activity. Perhaps you can color, read a story, or just snuggle close with your child or grandchild. Being selective with your time gives you the freedom to remove unnecessary "busy-ness" and focus on things that truly matter like tasting something good or smelling a freshly cut rose. People who live with life-threatening illnesses have said they can hear "the clock" ticking and time is getting away from them. Cancer patients learn many time management lessons and the most crucial one is to take time for the important things. You know what they are for you, and if you are unsure, consider this. "Yesterday is history, tomorrow is a mystery, today is a gift-that is why it is called the present" -Anonymous

≋*BREATHWORK & MEDITATION*

Breathwork is the general term used to describe many breathing techniques that are used in meditation and relaxation exercises. Deep breathing, such as breathing in through your nose and out through your mouth forcefully, is said to be cleansing to the body. The benefits of breathing properly are more than just physical, however; breathwork can help you release deep emotional wounds and painful feelings. Also known as breath therapy, it is a means of learning how to breathe consciously and fully to help with release of emotional pain. Ancient breathing techniques are found in the practices of yoga, t'ai chi, and qigong. These practices focus on breathing and the ability to transfer energy through the body and help you to connect with unexpressed emotions.

Meditation is a mind-body process that uses concentration or reflection to calm the mind and relax the body. It can help to reduce anxiety, lessen pain, lower blood pressure and heart rate, reduce stress, improve immune function, increase alertness, sharpen focus, raise self-awareness, improve mood, and create a general sense of well being. Other benefits of meditation are deeper relaxation, concentration on the present instead of the past and future, unconventional creativity, heightened spiritual awareness and a greater compassion for others and oneself as a whole. There are many approaches to meditation using different techniques, but most fall into one of three major categories:

transcendental meditation, which involves mental repetition of a mantra (a short affirmation or positive phrase); mindfulness meditation, which focuses on the present moment; and breath meditation, which calls for concentration on respiration (the process of inhaling and exhaling). Common to all forms of meditations are these requirements: a quiet environment, a comfortable position, and a point of focus for the mind. Most people prefer to keep their eyes closed to avoid visual distractions. Meditation can be self-directed or can be guided by mental health professionals, yoga masters, or doctors.

Here is a simple meditation technique that can be done almost anywhere and utilizes breathing to promote mental calmness: Select a quiet place and sit in a chair, with your back straight and your feet on the floor. Close your eyes and begin abdominal breathing, inhaling and exhaling through your nose at a rate of three to four full breaths (a breath = one inhalation and one exhalation) per minute. The object of this exercise is to stay focused on your breath, allowing whatever thoughts you have to come and go without being absorbed by them. Should you find your attention wandering, bring it back to your breath. You can also enhance the process by silently repeating a short affirmation, or a positive phrase, such as God, love, peace or white light, on both the inhalation and the exhalation. Try to do this exercise for five minutes once or twice a day, gradually working up to 20 minutes twice daily. Don't be discouraged if at first you find this exercise difficult to practice. It is not easy for most Americans to sit still and breathe without getting distracted or having some external stimulation. With time and continued practice, especially in the morning and before you go to bed, you will begin to notice the benefits meditation can give you. The longer you live with cancer as a chronic disease, the more likely you will be to need and appreciate the benefits of breathing, meditation and yoga. Meditation is like mental martial arts; you build up mental muscles of awareness in order to let go. It is a gentle growing process and is a way to enrich your life, bring peace to your heart and strengthen your mind. You should find your own personal method. Resources are available in libraries and bookstores. Meditation is a positive way of joining you together again with your Creator.

Terri – After undergoing major surgery, my sister was in excruciating pain that resulted in nausea and vomiting; she also had a gastric tube in her nose. We used meditation and breath work to help her through the pain; by doing this, she was able to stay focused on breathing and not on the tube down her throat. It is a controlled conscious effort to relax contracted muscles when immense pain is present. It was natural for her to hold her breath as most people do when in pain. By releasing the breath and allowing it to roll in and out continuously, you are letting go of the pain. You will notice this helps significantly.

≋ PERSONAL JOURNALING

Journaling provides the opportunity for you to record events occurring in your life as well as your feelings and emotional responses to those events. Writing what is significant to you at that time can serve as a healing tool. It can help you to identify thoughts, feelings, and behavior patterns. It allows you to observe what you are experiencing through a different lens – a recorded commentary of your experience.

Susan - When it was first suggested that I consider keeping a journal, I was quite skeptical about the process. After all, I am a woman who has trouble finishing a grocery list. I wasn't at all sure this was for me; however, I agreed to give it a try. I knew that to make an entry every day was totally unrealistic, so I decided to set aside time one day a week. I kept my journal by my bedside and would write in it first thing on Saturday morning. The lengths of my entries vary, and I find it is best for me if I just pick up the pen and start to write. Frequently, I am surprised by where my thought process leads me. At first, I was somewhat preoccupied with wondering how others would perceive my writing. I came to accept that sharing my thoughts would be strictly my choice and that allowed me a greater sense of freedom in what I recorded. In a few weeks, I found there were one or two recurrent themes to my entries. Being able to identify these themes helped me to put them in perspective and to better understand some of my feelings and responses regarding my journey with cancer. When I receive bad news, reviewing my journal helps me to compare my experiences with other difficult times.

Journaling is a wonderful coping mechanism. If you should decide to start journaling, the following suggestions may be helpful:

- Find a journal that is personal to you. It could be an attractive bound book or a simple spiral notebook. How it looks isn't important; what matters is that you have one place in which to keep your entries.
- If you need help starting, try writing, "I am thinking about..." or, "I was inspired by..." or, "I was surprised by..." or, "It touched my heart to..."

Don't worry about grammar or spelling; just go with the flow of your thoughts and feelings.

≋ SPECIAL PLACES FOR NURTURING THE SOUL

Do you have a "special place" that you feel drawn to in good times and bad, a place that brings you a sense of comfort and peace? It might be a path beside the lake, a stretch of beach by the ocean, a mountain view, a comfy chair that seems to fit you just right, or a place of worship. Perhaps your special place is not a physical location at all, but rather, a place where your mind can take you that brings you a sense of tranquility. Maybe your escape is an activity such as listening to music, working in the garden, or reading a good book. Whether the place is tangible or imaginary is not important. What matters is that you have discovered a comfort zone, where fears and worries can disappear. A retreat for a few minutes or a few hours can give you a sense of serenity. Dealing with cancer is very stressful, and you need to find a respite, however brief, from the harsh realities of the situation you have been given. Denial is not healthy; so acknowledge your stressful feelings, and try to identify ways to cope. Pick a place or experience that provides you with a sense of being cared for and refreshed so that you can maintain balance in your life. It is essential that you take time to nurture your soul. Discover or reconnect with whatever it is that brings you a sense of comfort and peace, and frequent that "special place." You will discover that it is time well spent.

≈ *WORK AND PLAY*

Is your job just a job or do you truly enjoy your chosen career? Are you fulfilled at the end of the day? Being unhappy in your work and the resulting stress it brings can rob you of your health. Your daily workplace is a vital aspect of your mental well-being. Even if you are fortunate enough to have a job you enjoy, you may not know how to relax completely at the end of the day. Are you subjecting yourself unnecessarily to the "dis-ease" of workaholism? It is essential that you regularly engage in the counterbalance to work – play. Many of us have associated playing with childhood; yet play is a crucial aspect of mental health and is unequaled in helping us express joy, passion, and exhilaration. The meaning of the word play is to dance, leap for joy, and rejoice - all activities that suggest a healthy mental state. Play has been described as any activity in which you lose track of time. Try to remember when you were a child, when things you did were pleasurable. Think of a special talent or gift you have, and use it to fill your heart with joy. Give yourself permission to play. If you have young children or pets at home, then you've already found the perfect playmates and a simple and wonderful way to become more childlike. Another option is to select a sport, dance, game, or other activity that requires you to move your body. Learn to play again!

CHAPTER ELEVEN

Spiritual Resources

✥ *ACTS OF LOVE –*

GIVING AND RECEIVING

Most of us are much more comfortable giving assistance than we are receiving it. Giving implies being in charge and having some control, while receiving assistance implies loss of control and can be most difficult to accept. You may find yourself on both sides of the equation at different times in the course of being a cancer patient. Focusing on the needs and concerns of someone else can be very healthful for you and the other person. Support and affirmation can give a person the courage to deal with adversity. Charity or altruism is helping others through donations of your time and resources and is not only spiritually rewarding but also, pleasurable.

Pam – I have come to understand over the years that sometimes all you can do for someone is listen with intention, and the blessing is, that just listening is enough.

Helping others with an open heart produces strong feelings of connection, a sense of unity, and the recognition that in giving to others you are ultimately giving to yourself. It is also a potent antidote for the negative effects of self-involvement. Learn to recognize your opportunities for altruism and take advantage of them.

Susan - I recall neighbors bringing dinner to our door numerous times during the course of recovering from surgeries and treatment. As much as I realized how helpful those dinners were for my family, it was hard to accept that I couldn't do it and needed others to assume that task. It was also hard for my husband who was very uncomfortable with the whole notion of having to receive charity. However, we did come to appreciate these acts for what they were – acts of kindness and concern on the part of others. Acts we would have gladly done for others had the roles been reversed. We came to realize that graciously accepting the kind help of others could also be a gift. We all have an innate need to connect with others and there is a value to the role of both the giver and the receiver. It actually became something of a joke in our family because it got so that when we would tell the kids that Mom had to go back into the hospital, after a few solicitous comments they would invariably ask "when will the good food start arriving?" So much for being in control of the kitchen!

We all have a desire to make a difference and we are each given an opportunity to do so. We simply need to develop the ability to identify those opportunities. As Mother Teresa said, "Few of us can do great things, but all of us can do small things with great love."

Nancy – Today I was reflecting on the power of love to heal. I think we learn how powerful love is in healing when we are small children. When you hurt yourself, your mother says, "let me kiss it and it will get better." – It's the first message that we get about love and healing. Love is a powerful healer!

🕊 *FAITH*

Some of the dictionary definitions of faith are: "confident belief; trust; belief in God; loyalty; allegiance."

Pam – Author Henry Nouwen writes about interviewing a famous circus performer and asking the trapeze flyer how he could perform such an extraordinary feat. The man told Nouwen that it was simple, that all he had to do was let go. The catcher does all the work. To me, that is the perfect definition of faith: just let go, and trust that God, the Great Catcher, will do all the work.

Faith is a sustaining force for many of us. Some individuals are able to explain clearly what their faith is, and while others may find it harder to define, this does not make life's spiritual aspects any less real or important to them. Faith brings an added dimension to our lives. It reaches beyond the concrete realities of our day-to-day situation and yet is an integral part of our daily existence. Our faith may be the result of a personal experience, the shared faith of another or we may regard it as the acceptance of a gift. We do not all share the same beliefs, but we do share the need to believe. It is not uncommon to re-examine our faith or beliefs during difficult times. If you were once a part of a faith community and have become distanced from it during the years, you may want to revisit those connections. Or perhaps you have always been active but are now questioning some of those beliefs about which you used to feel so sure. Just as you are gathering information and guidance about medical issues, remember to renew your connection in this important dimension of your life. There are many faith paths, and it is not for us to say we know what is right for you any more than we can prescribe your medical treatment. However, just as we have encouraged you to pursue your medical options and resources, we also encourage you in this area. Seek counsel from those in a position to assist you with your questions and uncertainties. Nurture the faith you have, whether it is a more formalized faith or a basic belief in mankind. Allow it to give you strength and to help you rejoice in the good things in life.

🕊 *FORGIVENESS*

Remember that you are a human being with imperfections, weaknesses, and flaws, like everyone else. Try to accept your mistakes and forgive yourself for them, canceling the demands that you *should have* behaved differently. Remove the guilt from your life; it is a useless torment. Do the same with others: forgive the person, not the action. Recognize your limitations, and also give yourself credit for all that you've achieved in spite of them. Doing so will allow you to be more accepting of yourself and others.

🕊 *GRATITUDE*

Most religious traditions practice specific prayers or grace before meals as a way of thanking God for your food and sustenance. As with other spiritual practices, there is something to be gained from these rituals, or they wouldn't have survived for thousands of years. A sense of gratitude for all the other areas of your life can bring forth similar life-enhancing benefits.

Nancy – This morning I woke up about 5am and the birds were singing so loudly and they sounded wonderful. As I listened, I kept thinking about a little blessing I learned as a child, which goes like this: Thank you for the food we eat; Thank you for the friends we meet; Thank you for the birds that sing; Thank you God for everything. Amen…That says it all in such a simple way.

Gratitude has been described as the "great attitude." Although most people tend to take their lives for granted, life is in fact a gift, and every day that you are alive you receive many blessings. Even times of pain and adversity can be seen as opportunities for growth for which you can be grateful. By committing yourself to becoming more aware of your blessings, you strengthen your connection with the Spirit and are better able to recognize the wisdom and intelligence that underlies all of creation. Once you allow yourself to appreciate the lessons presented during times of struggle or life crises, the brunt of the pain subsides and a state of inner peace follows. This is especially true of most chronic diseases, which sometimes can be seen as external reflections of inner (emotional and/or spiritual) pain. Typically, when people choose consciously to focus on the positives in their lives and express gratitude for them, more positive things start to happen. Gratitude can produce powerful feelings of joy and self-acceptance. It is an attitude that anyone can choose to have, just as you can choose to see the glass half-full or half-empty. By focusing on what you do have, instead of what you lack, you feel a sense of abundance and your problems seem much less severe; you are better able to let go of negative thoughts and attitudes. This usually isn't easy to do, especially if you are feeling a great deal of fear and anger. But if you make the effort to release these painful emotions and to choose the attitude of gratitude, even for a moment, wonderful things will begin to happen. Like any habit, recognizing and acknowledging the gifts in your life requires practice. One simple way to begin feeling grateful is the following visualization taught by Rabbi Mordecai Twerski, the spiritual leader of Denver's Hasidic community: As soon as you wake up each morning, before you get out of bed, close your eyes and picture a person, scene, or situation that made you happy to be alive and for which you are still grateful. You never would have had that experience if you weren't alive, and by allowing yourself to re-experience it, you open yourself up to the awareness that something equally wonderful can happen today. Create the habit of practicing this visualization each morning upon awakening, and you will soon instill in yourself a new attitude of anticipation and appreciation for the day ahead.

Another way to cultivate feelings of gratitude is by making a gratitude list. Think of every thing you have to be grateful for; even the smallest things can help you to appreciate your life, such as being able to read these words, having a chair to sit in, a bed to lie on, or food to eat. Complete the list by praying silently, giving thanks for all that you experienced and learned that day. By making gratitude a regular part of your daily experience, you set the stage for living more deeply connected to the Spirit. In the process, your life will be transformed into an increasingly joyous adventure.

🕊 *HOPE*

Optimism and hope are radically different attitudes. Optimism is the expectation that things – the weather, human relationships, the economy, the political situation, and so on – will get better. Hope is the trust that God will fulfill His promises to us in a way that leads us to true freedom. The optimist speaks about concrete changes in the future. The person of hope lives in the moment with the knowledge and trust that all of life is in good hands. All the great spiritual leaders in history were people of hope; Abraham, Moses, Ruth, Mary, Jesus, Buddha, Mohammed, and Gandhi all lived with a promise in their hearts that guided them toward the future without the need to know exactly what it would look like. Make a choice to live with hope.

Nancy – I know that I would much rather die with hope than to live with hopelessness. Hope gives us the spark to help us live each day to the fullest. Don't let anyone steal your hope. There may not be another treatment available, but there is something that can be done to make our lives better while our scientists struggle to find the cure. There is always hope.

🕊 *PRAYER*

Prayer is the most common form of spiritual exercise. Nearly 90 percent of people pray, and 70 percent believe that prayer can lead to physical, emotional, and spiritual healing. When you pray you can have a greater sense of well-being, and through prayer you can experience a sense of peace, receive answers to life issues, and may feel divinely inspired or "led by God" to perform some specific action. People who experience a "sense of the Divine" during prayer also report a sense of general well-being and satisfaction in their lives. Many studies are now being done to prove scientifically that prayer makes a difference in the healing process and in a person's overall well-being. Some studies have shown that those people who are prayed for recover faster and have less pain. Prayer not only helps the patient, but it is also beneficial to those who are doing the praying. Dr. Herbert Benson of Harvard reports that repetitive prayer and non-religious meditation have very similar relaxation effects, but that people find more emotional comfort in prayer. Repetitive prayer slows a person's heartbeat and breathing rate, lowers blood pressure, and calms brain waves without drugs. To begin the practice of prayer, start with any prayer you are comfortable with or that you recall from your religious training as a child. You can also use a favorite Psalm or other passage from the Bible or prayer book you find especially meaningful. In addition, you can engage in personal prayer, talking to God as if you were speaking to your best friend. State your need or concern and ask for God's help; it is more rewarding to pray for the peace that would result from having what you desire than for the specific things themselves. Whichever form of prayer you choose, try to establish a regular routine and repeat your prayer morning and night. A meaningful prayer for all of us has been to ask God to do according to His will that which is for our highest and best good.

Nancy's Prayer – Dear God, as I walk through this life, the culmination of my journey is to be with You. Help me to remember that You are always holding my hand as I take each step; that You are guiding me every step of the way. Some of these steps may be joyous and buoyant, filled with good health and happiness and some may be filled with pain – either from illness, loss, misunderstandings and other challenges in my path. You have promised that You are always with me, that Your peace will always be with me as I travel on my journey. Help me to learn from every experience I face on this journey. Give me the courage I need to face the unknown and the knowledge to know the meaning of the lessons in my life. As I walk through this journey of life, I am comforted to know that Your rod and staff will prevent me from stumbling; Your goodness and mercy will follow me every day of my life and Your peace will comfort me in sickness and in health. Your healing hand will deliver me from earthly pain if it becomes more than I can bear.

Thank You for every opportunity I have to let a light shine through me to help others on their pathway. Whatever the test, I rest in the knowledge that You are always there and You will always take care of me and those I love. Thank you for guiding and loving me.   AMEN

God be in my head and in my understanding;

God be in my eyes and in my looking;

God be in my mouth and in my speaking;

God be in my heart and in my thinking;

God be at my end and in my departing.

Sarum Primer 1538.

Serenity Prayer

God grant me the serenity to accept the things I cannot change;

The courage to change the things I can;

And the wisdom to know the difference.

Living one day at a time;

Enjoying one moment at a time;

Accepting hardships as the pathway to peace;

Taking, as He did, this sinful world as it is, not as I would have it;

Trusting that He will make all things right if I surrender to His will;

That I may be reasonably happy in this life

and supremely happy with Him;

Forever in the next.

Amen

Reinhold Neibuhr

PART VI - Upstaging

CHAPTER TWELVE

Surviving Stage IV and

Thriving at Stage V

RECURRENCE

After your initial bout with cancer, the thought of recurrence stays with you for a long time. You want believe it is over and that you won't ever have to experience this dreaded disease again. Being re-diagnosed is a serious blow to even the strongest survivor. However, because you have been down this road before, you are able to lean upon a base of knowledge that was acquired through past experience. You are already familiar with the doctors, nurses, treatment facilities and terminology. You may not want to go through treatment again, but you know that life is still calling you to live.

Nancy – I think about cancer like it is a sandcastle. All at once we hear the word, cancer, and our world is torn apart – like a sandcastle washed away by the waves. We think our dreams are shattered. We can't believe the world is going along as if all is well when our life has been crushed. The lesson I've learned is when cancer shatters one's life, just remember you can build again. With each recurrence, you can build again. Don't let it crush you. You can build again!

LIVING WITH CANCER AS A CHRONIC DISEASE

For some patients the cancer road is much longer; it continues from recurrence to recurrence. Countless people are surviving and living with cancer as a chronic disease for many years. Your life has changed dramatically, but you can expect this change to become easier with each passing day. Your focus will shift from keeping the disease under control to maintaining a satisfying lifestyle. You will always be in search of that perfect drug that will cure you, and every day will be a challenge. There will be days that you want to quit, but you can't stop living. You know that no one is going to live forever, but you also know that your chances of living as long as other people are limited. You have an opportunity to look at life differently now. It is now that you start living your <u>real</u> life – thanking God for this new awareness - seeing things as you have never seen them before: watching God's pallet as he paints the sunset, the brilliance of stars in the night sky, seeing the many colors of spring in bloom, hearing a bluebird singing just for you, and looking at your children and grandchildren in precious new ways. Your priorities, your perspectives, everything will change. You have heightened awareness of everything. You learn to let go of your limitations and inhibitions; there's a new freedom to living, and a freedom from other people's expectations. You realize that what someone thinks of you can't give one you extra day of living.

There's no amount of money that can buy you a longer life.

Terri – I don't think people realize that living with cancer is not a tragedy; it's actually a blessing because I can see life in a different light. I wake up every day and God continues to give me the will to live. He encourages me to fill the spirit of my soul and share that spirit with others.

Nancy –I grew up on a farm in the mountains of North Carolina near West Jefferson, and we had several fruit trees. I learned that if a tree stops bearing that you could cut a gash in the tree and for some unknown reason that tree will begin to bear fruit again. I think the gash is a wake-up call to us to examine our lives and see what we are doing to be fruitful.

Try to use this time to look inward and know that you have it within your power to make your life meaningful to yourself and others.

Nancy – Focus on things that are uplifting to you, not draining. If a relationship is draining, don't foster it. If your job is not giving you joy, find ways that you can find joy in it or figure out a way to change it or change jobs.

Living courageously with this disease is a powerful example to others who are facing this difficult diagnosis. When you realize that you will be living with cancer as a chronic illness, use the knowledge gained from your experience as an opportunity to help others. No one gets the luxury of selecting life's problems, but how you deal with them makes all the difference.

Three of us have experienced living at Stage IV with cancer. We know that we have been blessed to choose what we do with the privileged time given. New treatment options are developed everyday, and researchers with fresh ideas are graduating and just beginning to put their talents to work.

Susan – My journey as a cancer patient these past 23 years has been like a game of lost and found...I thought I would never again feel at peace, experience joy or believe that life is good. But instead...I found the wonder of appreciating just how precious life is and learned to look upon each day as a gift. I found the pleasure of seeing myself as a truly unique individual and stopped trying to be just like everyone else. I found the incredible freedom that comes with realizing that I am not in control, I am not in charge. I found that there are many ways to applaud life, give hugs and make peanut butter sandwiches, that don't require two hands. I found the peace that comes from within, the joy of experiencing God's love and His gift of love from others and I found that life is good. In this game of lost and found, I have come to realize I have found much more than I have lost.

We all are more likely to say, "I love you," laugh at corny jokes, and discover beauty where we least expect it. We choose to remain hopeful and nurture our spirits while tending to our physical needs. Strive for the healing of your mind - body - spirit.

It is important that you not only survive this experience, but also learn to thrive -- not so much in spite of it, but as a result of it. It is not a life path that you would have chosen, but it is one that can enrich your life beyond measure.

*Nancy – My body hasn't been cured, but cancer has truly been a healing experience for my life. Cure and healing are not the same. One can be perfectly healthy, and not have a life that is healed. Your goal should be to focus on healing your life and how you do that depends upon your individual needs. Listen to your inner voice and you will know what you need to heal your life. It may be to mend a dispute, get more exercise, diet, or to get in touch with your spiritual side. If you are holding grudges, let them go because by holding on you are giving someone else control over your life and it affects your health. Forgive yourself and others and heal your heart. Whatever it is, listen to that still, small voice and follow that guidance. When you focus on healing your life, who knows?-- your disease may be cured in the meantime because you are feeding your soul. **I know there is a difference between healing and being cured – healing lasts an eternity.***

Epilogue

Our dear friends, Nancy Emerson and Susan Moonan, completed their cancer journeys during the course of writing this book. Although they were never cured of this disease, both their lives were healed as completely as any we have ever known. They lived every day with hope and joy, which has served as inspiration for all who knew them. It was their fondest wish to be able to offer help and comfort to those of you who travel this same difficult journey. They would want you to be inspired by their lives that defied all statistics, confounded experts, and amazed and empowered friends and loved ones. They were living miracles whose lives transformed so many who were privileged to be touched by them. It is our hope that their lives will continue to light the path for others through their wisdom and hard-learned lessons documented in this book. We rejoice in our opportunity to share with you some of their advice, hope and encouragement, added to our own.

May you be lifted up by the love and light that sustain us.

Acknowledgements

We would like to acknowledge everyone who contributed to the content of this book, especially Amma, Clarice Davis, for the many meals she prepared, for keeping the dogs busy while we worked and for her loving encouragement of our work in progress. We would also like to thank our husbands, Johnny Emerson, George Leight, George Moonan and Eric Schinazi, for their love, patience and support. We especially appreciate the help of Melanie Leight, Rita Deimler, Kathy Becker, Gail Funk, Georgie Dacuycuy, Leigh and Bill Kempf, Ann Hubbard, Peter Winkler and Harriet Ballard for their contributions. We are grateful to the cancer patients who offered their advice, tips and stories; and to Kelly Marcom, MD, for his incomparable care, concern, and friendship and for writing our Foreword.

Tree of Life cover art by Terri Schinazi

Resources

BOOKS

A HELPING HAND, The Resource Guide for People with Cancer, Cancer
  Care Inc., 2002, 275 Seventh Ave. NY NY 10001, 800-813-HOPE (4673)
  E-mail - info@cancercare.org

BREAD FOR THE JOURNEY, A Daybook of Wisdom and Faith, Henri J. M.
  Nouwen, HarperCollins, San Francisco, 1997.

THE COMPLETE SELF-CARE GUIDE TO HOLISTIC MEDICINE, Robert
  S. Ivker, D.O., Tarcher/Putnam, 1999.

COPING WITH CHEMOTHERAPY, Nancy Bruning, Avery Press, August
  2002.

DR. GAYNOR'S CANCER PREVENTION PROGRAM, Mitchell l. Gaynor,
  MD, Kensington Health, 1999.

EATING WELL FOR OPTIMUM HEALTH, Andrew Weil, MD., Alfred A.
  Knopf, Random House, New York, 2000.

THE HEALING POWER OF FAITH – HOW BELIEF AND PRAYER CAN
  HELP YOU TRIUMPH OVER DISEASE, Harold G. Koenig, M.D., Duke
  University

NATIONAL CANCER INSTITUTE AND CANCERNET

Most clinics have pamphlets available about different types of cancer. You
  may also obtain free pamphlets by calling the National Cancer Institute at
  1-800-4-CANCER to request them.

When Someone in Your Family Has Cancer - Children's Book available from
  the NCI – 800-422-6237.

NATURAL HEALTH, NATURAL MEDICINE, Andrew Weil, M.D.,
  Houghton Mifflin, 215 Park Avenue South, NYNY 10003,1995.

SEXUALITY & CANCER, American Cancer Society, Leslie R. Schover,
  Ph.D., American Cancer Society, 1988, Free 1-800-ACS-2345

YOU CAN'T AFFORD THE LUXURY OF A NEGATIVE THOUGHT, The
  Life 101 Series, Peter McWilliams, Prelude Press, 1988.

FINANCIAL HELP

Patient Access Network Foundation – 1-866-316-7263
  www.patientaccessnetwork.org

Healthwell Foundation 1-800-675-8416

Resources

www.healthwellfoundation.org

Patient Advocate Foundation's Co-Pay Relief Program 1-866-512-3861

www.copays.org

Patient Services Incorporated 1-800-366-7741

www.uneedpsi.org

National Organization for Rare Disorders 1-203-744-0100

www.rarediseases.org

Partnership for Prescription Assistance 1-888-477-2669

www.pparx.org

Cancer Care

www.cancercare.org

Government Benefits or Entitlements

- Social Security Disability, Supplemental Security Income, and Medicare benefits: 1-800-772-1213, or www.ssa.gov
- Medicare and Medicaid: 1-877-267-2323 www.cms.hhs.gov
- Food Stamps and public assistance: 1-877-696-6675 or www.os.dhhs.gov
- National Energy Assistance Referral: 1-866-674-6327

INFORMATION HOTLINES

Alliance for Lung Cancer Advocacy - 800-298-2436

American Amputee Foundation, Inc. –501-666-9560 (toll)

American Brain Tumor Association – 800-886-2282

American Cancer Society – 800-227-2345

American Chronic Pain Association – 703-648-8912 (toll)

American Liver Foundation – 800-223-0179

American Lung Association – 800-LUNG-USA

Bone & Marrow Transplant Information Network
    847-433-3313 (toll)

Cancer Care, Inc. – 800-813-4673

Cancer Hope Network – 877-467-3638

Cancer Information Service (NCI)– 800-422-6237

Kids Count Too! (ACS) – 800-227-2345

Kids Konnected – 800-899-2866

Resources

National Women's Health Information Center (NWHIC)

    800-994-9662 English/Spanish

    888-220-5446 TDD

Susan G. Komen Breast Cancer Foundation's 1-800-I'M

    AWARE Helpline – 800-462-9273

Gilda's Club Worldwide – 888-445-3248

The Wellness Community – 888-793-9355

MAGAZINES

COPING MAGAZINE - $18.00/one year subscription, 1-615-791-3859

CURE (Cancer Updates, Research & Education) Free to cancer patients and survivors, $20.00/one year subscription, Cancer Information Group, LP, 3535 Worth St., Collins Tower, Ste 185, Dallas, TX 75246, visit www.curetoday.com

PROFESSIONAL ASSOCIATIONS

The American Society of Clinical Oncology (ASCO)

1900 Duke Street, Suite 200

Alexandria, VA 22314

(703) 299-0150

www.asco.org   www.peoplelivingwithcancer.org

ASCO is an organization that represents more than 18,000 cancer professionals worldwide. The ASCO site has a search index that can help you easily locate topics, such as clinical trials, local resources, etc.

The Association of Oncology Social Work (AOSW)

4700 W. Lake Ave.

Glenview, IL 60025

(847) 375-4721

www.aosw.org

AOSW is a non-profit, international organization dedicated to the enhancement of psychosocial services to people with cancer and their families. The AOSW site provides links to oncology resources like cancer information, organizations, cancer centers and disease-specific sites for adults and children.

The Oncology Nursing Society (ONS)

Resources

501 Holiday Drive

Pittsburgh, PA 15220

(412) 921-7373

www.ons.org

ONS is a national organization of more than 30,000 registered nurses and other
health care professionals dedicated to patient care, teaching, research,
administration, and education in the field of oncology.

WEBSITES

The internet is a great source of cancer information, but you will find that all
websites are not equally reliable. To avoid getting lots of useless data, you
should be as specific as possible when you enter your search topic. Your
physician or members of your healthcare team may be able to suggest some
other reliable websites. Below is a list of the websites that should fill your
major resource needs.

Government Sites

NATIONAL CANCER INSTITUTE

www.icic.nci.nih.gov The National Institute of Health (NIH) government
sponsored site, which provides access to information statements from the
National Cancer Institute's Physician Data Query (PDQ) database, fact
sheets on various cancer topics and services provided by the Cancer
Information Service, which can also be reached by phone at 800-4-
CANCER.

wwwcancernet.nci.nih.gov CancerNet

wwwclinicaltrials.gov (NIH) Clinical Trials

www.nlm.nih.gov (NIH) US National Library of Medicine

www.cancer.gov/espanol (Spanish information)

www.cancer.gov (search site using full title) CANCER TRIALS – 10
Things to Know about Evaluating Medical Resources on the Web

ASSOCIATION OF CANCER ONLINE RESOURCES

www.acor.org

BREAST CANCER RESOURCE DIRECTORY OF NORTH CAROLINA

www.bcresourcedirectory.org

CANCER CARE, INC.

Resources

www.cancercare.org

www.cancercare.org/espanol/index.asp (Spanish)

CANCER PREVENTION PROGRAM

www.gaynoroncology.com

CANCER RESEARCH & PREVENTION FOUNDATION

www.preventcancer.org

Clinics and Research Centers

Johns Hopkins Oncology Center

www.hopkinscancercenter.org

Dana-Farber Cancer Institute

www.dana-farber.net

Duke Comprehensive Cancer Center

www.cancer.duke.edu

Mayo Clinic Cancer Center

www.mayo.edu/MayoHome.html

MD Anderson Cancer Center

www.mdanderson.org

Memorial Sloan Kettering Cancer Center

www.mskcc.org/mskee/html/44.cfm

AGING WITH DIGNITY

www.agingwithdignity.com

AMERICAN CANCER SOCIETY

www.acs.org

CONSUMER LAB

www.consumerlab.com

CORPORATE ANGELS NETWORK, INC.

www.corpangelnetwork.org

CAN finds free air transportation (on corporate planes) for cancer patients
who need medical treatments. (Patients must be ambulatory).

GILDA'S CLUB WORLDWIDE

www.gildasclub.org

HOSPICE EDUCATION INSTITUTE

www.hospiceworld.org

Resources

KID'S CANCER NETWORK

    www.kidscancernetwork.org

LEUKEMIA & LYMPHOMA SOCIETY

    www.leukemia-lymphoma.org

MAKE-A-WISH FOUNDATION OF AMERICA

    www.wish.org

MEDICALERT®

    www.medicalert.org

MEDINFO.ORG

    www.cure.medinfo.org

    Provides a list of cancer discussion groups, home pages written by cancer survivors and links to other cancer sites.

NATIONAL CENTER FOR COMPLEMENTARY AND ALTERNATIVE MEDICINE

    wwwnncam.nia.gov

NATIONAL COALITION OF CANCER SURVIVORSHIP

    www.cansearch.org - Survivorship-Spirituality Program

NATIONAL FAMILY CAREGIVERS ASSOCIATION

    www.nfcacares.org

ONCOLINK

    www.oncolink.com (search under "listserv")

PATIENT ADVOCATE FOUNDATION

    www.patientadvocate.org

    Provides cancer patients with help dealing with insurance coverage, paying for managed care and offers legal intervention for insurance issues through a National Legal Resources Network.

QUACKWATCH

    www.quackwatch.com A non-profit site founded to expose cases of heath fraud on the web.

R.A. BLOCH - REFERRAL SITE

    www.blastcancer.org The Richard and Annette Bloch Cancer Foundation Second Opinion Referral centers in the United States.

SOCIAL SECURITY ADMINISTRATION (Disability)

Resources

www.ssa.gov

UNIVERSITY OF PENNSYLVANIA CANCER LINKS

www.cancer.med.upenn.edu Developed and maintained through the Univ.
of Pennsylvania, this site contains links to educational information and
supportive resource sites on the Web.

WebMD

www.Webmd.com

WIGS

www.headcovers.com

Y-ME

www.y-me.org

Index

Index

Index

Index

Index

Index

Index

Notes

Notes

Notes

Notes

Notes
